TORRANCE PUBLIC LIBRARY

3 2111 01133 4890

W9-BSN-562

KATY GEISSERT
CIVIC CENTER LIBRARY

WITHDRAWN

# WHEN GERMS TRAVEL

A Chicago Tribune Book of the Year

"A critically important book for this historical moment. . . . A clarion call for the public (and the government) to recognize both the importance and the precariousness of public health as we enter the twenty-first century." —*Health Affairs*

"Deft, interesting and informative." —*The Roanoke Times*

"Dr. Markel is an epic historian, a wise scientist, and an elegant prose stylist. . . . Written with humor, grace, insight, and warmth, *When Germs Travel* is a discerning portrait of illness, a comment on the immigrant experiences of the past and present, and a reflection on what it means to be a doctor in a society ruled by fear of contagion."
—Andrew Solomon, author of *The Noonday Demon*

"Markel writes with great attention to the human side of the story. . . . A powerful, sweeping story about immigration, poverty, public health, scientific breakthroughs and medical failures." —*Chicago Free Press*

"Markel proves just how compelling medical history can be in these lucid, thought-provoking accounts of the complex intersection of immigration policy and public health."
—Andrea Barrett, author of *Ship Fever*

"Highly readable. . . . Dramatic and graphic."
—*Tucson Citizen*

"A timely book. Markel, a medical historian and himself a physician, knows that the so-called general reader needs to be guided through the maze of technicalities, and he does the guiding in a text as readable as it is reliable. It reads like a thriller."
—Peter Gay, Sterling Professor of History Emeritus, Yale University

"Solid information on a serious subject, delivered with great assurance and style."                    —*Kirkus Reviews*

"Dr. Markel . . . is both passionate and compassionate about his subject and conveys this devotion in clear, precise, gentle prose that is in the tradition of such great doctor-writers as A. J. Cronin, Somerset Maugham, Sherwin Nuland, Lewis Thomas, and William Carlos Williams—doctors for whom the patient was the important part of the story most necessary for breaking the reader's heart."
                    —Larry Kramer, author of *Reports from the Holocaust*

"A crisp, brisk and matter-of-fact narrative that can be more chilling than anything Stephen King has ever committed to paper. . . . This important cautionary tale proves infectiously readable."                    —*Flint Journal*

"Informative and important. . . . For each epidemic, Markel weaves a vivid description of the natural history of the disease with an account of how the disease entered the United States, spread and ultimately faded away. Markel portrays these events through engrossing stories of individual victims. . . . Enthralling. His ability to make medicine accessible and understandable to lay readers is remarkable."
                    —*St. Louis Post-Dispatch*

"In this very readable book, Markel chronicles yet another way in which this fear has played a critical role in the history of the U.S.—a nation built from collections of others. In addition to telling a fascinating historical story . . . this book reminds us all that prejudice, no less than science, often drives health policy."                    —*Jerusalem Post*

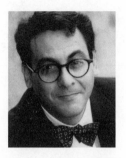

*Howard Markel*

# WHEN GERMS TRAVEL

Howard Markel is the George E. Wantz Professor of the History of Medicine and Professor of Pediatrics and Communicable Diseases at the University of Michigan, where he directs the Center for the History of Medicine. He is the author of the award-winning *Quarantine!* and numerous articles for scholarly publications, as well as for *The New York Times*, *Harper's*, *The Atlantic Monthly*, *The Washington Post*, and National Public Radio.

ALSO BY HOWARD MARKEL

AUTHOR

*Quarantine!: East European Jewish Immigrants
and the New York City Epidemics of 1892*

COAUTHOR

*The H. L. Mencken Baby Book*

*The Portable Pediatrician*

*The Practical Pediatrician: The A to Z Guide to
Your Child's Health, Behavior, and Safety*

COEDITOR

*Formative Years: Children's Health in the United States, 1880–2000*

# WHEN GERMS TRAVEL

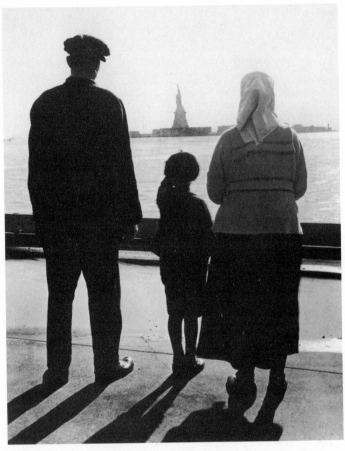

*An immigrant family looks at the Statue of Liberty as they await the barge that will take them from Ellis Island to their new lives in America.*

614.49
M345

# WHEN GERMS TRAVEL

Six Major Epidemics That Have Invaded America
and the Fears They Have Unleashed

KGL

# HOWARD MARKEL

Vintage Books
A Division of Random House, Inc.
New York

FIRST VINTAGE BOOKS EDITION, MAY 2005

*Copyright © 2004 by Howard Markel*

All rights reserved under International and Pan-American Copyright Conventions.
Published in the United States by Vintage Books, a division of Random House, Inc., New
York, and simultaneously in Canada by Random House of Canada Limited, Toronto.
Originally published in hardcover in the United States by Pantheon Books, a division of
Random House, Inc., New York, in 2004.

Vintage and colophon are registered trademarks of Random House, Inc.

The Library of Congress has cataloged the Pantheon edition as follows:
Markel, Howard.
When germs travel : six major epidemics that have invaded America and
the fear they have unleashed / Howard Markel.
p.   cm
Includes index.
1. Communicable diseases—United States—History—19th century.   2. Communicable
diseases—United States—History—20th century.   3. Epidemics—United States—
History—19th century.   4. Epidemics—United States—History—20th century.   I. Title.
RC111.M226 2004
614.4'973—dc22
2003062325

**Vintage ISBN: 0–375–72602–0**

*Author photograph © Joyce Ravid*
*Book design by Iris Weinstein*

www.vintagebooks.com

Printed in the United States of America
10   9   8   7   6   5   4   3   2   1

*To Kate,*
*who makes everything in my life, both on and off the written page, better*

# CONTENTS

# ILLUSTRATIONS

Frontispiece. Immigrants at Ellis Island. Library of Congress.

Page 11. Dr. William Carlos Williams. Back cover of *The Autobiography of William Carlos Williams* (New York: Random House, 1951).

Page 17. Louis Pasteur. From *Vanity Fair*, Jan. 8, 1887. Collections of the University of Michigan Center for the History of Medicine.

Page 29. Robert Koch. Collections of the University of Michigan Center for the History of Medicine.

Page 33. "Don't Kiss Me!" WPA poster, circa 1936. Collections of the University of Michigan Center for the History of Medicine.

Page 37. Saranac Tuberculosis Sanatorium. Collections of the University of Michigan Center for the History of Medicine.

Page 50. Chinatown, San Francisco, circa 1890s. Collections of the University of Michigan Center for the History of Medicine.

Page 57. Immigrants being vaccinated for smallpox, 1904. Library of Congress.

Page 63. Chinatown, San Francisco, circa 1900–1901. Collections of the University of Michigan Center for the History of Medicine.

Page 75. A Chinese greengrocer, Chinatown, San Francisco, circa 1900–1901. Collections of the University of Michigan Center for the History of Medicine.

Page 82. Ellis Island, 1902. From "Quarantine Sketches," promotional brochure. Collections of the University of Michigan Center for the History of Medicine.

# AUTHOR'S NOTE

With the exception of Chick Gin, Rabbi Chaim Goldenbaum, and Carmelita Torres (whose stories were reported in newspapers during their lifetimes), the names and some of the identifying features of the immigrant patients presented on these pages have been altered. It should also be noted that "Tomás," who appears in Chapter Five, actually represents a composite of two Haitian refugees.

# ACKNOWLEDGMENTS

Although the writing of a book is a solitary act, its transformation into a volume that you can actually hold in your hands and read is very much a group effort. I have been most fortunate over the past seven years because of the support of many foundations, institutions, friends, and colleagues.

I received generous financial support to research and write this book from the Robert Wood Johnson Foundation (in the form of a Generalist Faculty Scholars Award), the National Institutes of Health (the James A. Shannon Director's Award), and the Burroughs-Wellcome Fund (the 40th Anniversary History of Medicine Award).

I am grateful to Dr. Karen Brudney of the Tuberculosis Clinic of New York–Presbyterian Hospital for allowing me to interview some of her patients; to Lynne Partington, former director, her staff, and the residents of Freedom House in Detroit; and the staffs of the National Archives Records Administration, the University of Michigan Libraries, the Library of Congress, the American Jewish Historical Society, YIVO Institute for Jewish Studies, the New York Academy of Medicine, and the National Library of Medicine. An earlier version of Chapter Three appeared in the *Bulletin of the History of Medicine* 74 (2000): 525–60. When discussing the typhus and cholera epidemics of 1892, I used six paragraphs from my previous book, *Quarantine!*. I thank the Johns Hopkins University Press for permission to incorporate these materials into the text.

During the 1999–2000 academic year, I had the honor of being an Inaugural Fellow at the Dorothy and Lewis Cullman Center for Scholars and Writers at the New York Public Library. Aside from spending a glorious year in an office overlooking the majestic lions, Patience and Fortitude, I benefited greatly from the intellectual stimulation and support of my "fellow fellows," especially Andrew Delbanco, Ada Louise Huxtable, Allen Kurzweil, Francine Prose, and Harvey Sachs. I am also indebted to the Center's director emeritus, Peter Gay, the Library's president, Paul LeClerc, and the superb staff of the New York Public Library.

At the University of Michigan, I am fortunate to have several caring and inspiring colleagues who reviewed the manuscript and helped me to improve it, including Professors Horace Davenport, Nicholas Delbanco, Janet Gilsdorf, Frederick Neidhardt, Michael Schoenfeldt, Alexandra Minna Stern, and Arthur Vander. A special acknowledgment must be made to my dean, Dr. Allen S. Lichter, who has been instrumental in making the University of Michigan Medical School a welcome academic home for me.

Other colleagues who took time from their work to help me clarify my ideas include Susan Abrams of the Johns Hopkins Institute of the History of Medicine; Andrea Barrett; Dr. Joseph Cook, president emeritus of the International Trachoma Initiative; Professor Bert Hansen at Baruch College, City University of New York; Christopher Meehan, my former research assistant; Professor David Rosner at Columbia University; Professor Walton O. Schalick III of Washington University; Marian Smith, senior historian of the U.S. Immigration and Naturalization Service; and Professor Abraham Verghese of the University of Texas at San Antonio.

My literary agents, Glen Hartley and Lynn Chu, were involved in this project from the very beginning, and I have benefited so much from their creativity, intelligence, expertise, and support.

My editor, Victoria Wilson, vice president and associate publisher of Alfred A. Knopf, is nothing short of extraordinary. She held me to the highest standards of writing, and her wise suggestions and advice made this book far better than it would have otherwise been.

Finally, there are two women in my life whom I am most grateful to acknowledge: my wonderful daughter, Bess, and my lovely wife, Kate. But with all due respect to Bess, who at three cannot yet read, every line of this book was carefully scrutinized and typically improved by her very literate mother. Alas, any errors or omissions in this book rest solely on my shoulders.

HOWARD MARKEL
*Ann Arbor, Michigan*
*September 17, 2003*

# WHEN GERMS TRAVEL

# INTRODUCTION

And if a stranger sojourn with thee in your land, you shall not vex him. But the stranger that dwelleth with you shall be unto you as one born among you, and thou shall love him as thyself; for you were strangers in the land of Egypt.

— LEVITICUS[1]

Infectious disease is one of the great tragedies of living things—the struggle for existence between different forms of life. Man sees it from his own prejudiced point of view; but clams, oysters, insects, fish, flowers, tobacco, potatoes, tomatoes, fruit, shrubs, trees, have their own varieties of smallpox, measles, cancer, or tuberculosis. Incessantly, the pitiless war goes on, without quarter or armistice—a nationalism of species against species.

— HANS ZINSSER, M.D., *Rats, Lice and History*[2]

Our struggle against deadly microbes is endless. Scourges that have plagued human beings since the ancients still threaten to unleash themselves; new maladies are brewing that have yet to make their appearance in the headlines; and lethal germs employed as weapons of warfare and terrorism have again emerged as a worldwide menace. Some germs kill rapidly; others are able to live within their hosts for lengthy periods causing chronic disease. Regardless of their mode of attack or cohabitation, microbes exist solely to multiply, thrive, and find new hosts. The most egalitarian of living organisms, they cross all national boundaries and every social class, attacking without prejudice. Simply put, germs travel.

Not surprisingly, human beings are among the most common vectors of epidemic disease. As humans travel, so, too, do the infections we may harbor. Increasingly, globalization, social upheaval, and international travel render us all potential inhabitants of the so-called Hot Zone. How ironic, then, that the United States, a country which has prided itself since inception on being a nation of immigrants, continues its lengthy tradition of blaming newcomers for many of its physical and social ills. Today, more than two-thirds of all Americans are either immigrants themselves or the children or grandchildren of immigrants.[3] The experiences of moving great distances from one nation and culture to another, anxieties over adapting to the "American way of life," and stigmatization because of one's foreign appearance, accent, or manners are still fresh memories or everyday realities for many millions of newcomers who have made America their home. Still, the association of immigrants with imported infections remains, and stories of their journeys, illnesses, and treatment reveal much about our predispositions for dealing with the perpetual threat of contagious disease.

This book began out of my work as an AIDS physician during the late 1980s and early 1990s. At the time I was enrolled in graduate school for a Ph.D. in medical history, and my clinical and scholarly work enjoyed a mutually beneficial relationship microbiologists might call symbiotic. Every Monday and Wednesday evening for three years, I saw dozens of patients, mostly young gay men and intravenous drug users, with HIV or AIDS. I became especially intrigued by a question that kept popping up during our conversations: "Dr. Markel, do you think I will be quarantined because I have AIDS?" Doctors rarely hear the same question from so many different patients, but when they do they listen carefully. During these encounters I learned that long before coming to the clinic, my patients experienced many forms of stigmatization that affected their lives and health care. Their fear of being isolated on a distant island by some social edict or legal action did not seem all that great a leap.

I was troubled by these conversations and began to explore the history of the quarantine in American society. One hot summer afternoon, while in the stacks of the library, I stumbled onto the 1892 annual report of the New York City Department of Health. Its pages describe in great detail two deadly epidemics, cholera and typhus fever, that resulted in the strict isolation of the Eastern European Jewish immigrants who physically imported both infections into the United States. Thus began my initial venture in documenting the episodic collisions of immigrants and epidemic disease in America.[4]

During the late nineteenth century, physicians had little to offer in treating or preventing epidemic diseases, and the quarantine of those discovered to be ill was one of the few means available. There were, on the other hand, a few factors working in favor of these doctors in 1892. In the case of cholera, the ten-day transatlantic voyages gave the disease enough time to declare itself among most of the infected immigrants, affording the physicians an opportunity to isolate those passengers upon arrival. With the typhus fever epidemic, which had a much longer incubation period than cholera, most of the victims traveled on the same steamship and were residing temporarily in six boardinghouses on the Lower East Side of New York City. This scenario made the search for typhus a relatively simple (albeit panic-stricken) affair. The strategy in both cases was obvious: to draw a line of separation around those who were deemed to be ill or harboring infection—the newly arrived immigrants.

My attraction to these particular newcomers, undoubtedly, had its roots in my own background as the grandchild of East European Jewish immigrants. The sounds of Yiddish filled our household; indeed, as a child, I quickly realized that all the really interesting conversations were in the *mama-loshen* (mother tongue), so I worked hard to develop some facility with it. Still, it took me many more years to appreciate how disruptive the immigration experience was to the lives and psyches of my grandparents and others like them. They were, as described by Ruth Gay, truly "unfinished people" who desperately wanted to be accepted by their newly adopted land but were more often held back by their foreign accents and sensibilities and an unhealthy dose of fear.[5] While they certainly assimilated into American life as best they could, a generation or two of finishing was required before their progeny would blend in, ever mindful of the both comforting and suffocating warmth of *Yiddishkeit.*

Of all the maladies that strike human beings, I have chosen to document those of the contagious variety, germs that travel from one living being to another, because there is a narrative power to the epidemics they can cause. These events typically unfold dramatically and contain elements of discovery, reaction, suspense, conflict, illness, perhaps death, and, one hopes, resolution. Yet both history and recent experience teach us that, in most cases, the conclusions of these episodes are flat and anticlimactic; public health crises typically fade away with what one historian has described as "a whimper rather than a bang."[6] Too often, epidemics conclude with a return to a similar set of social and public health conditions that may have given rise to them in the first place.

In the decades that followed the 1892 epidemics, the relationship between human beings and microbes changed with scientific advances in our understanding and amelioration of infectious diseases. Over the past fifty years in particular, with the advent of miraculous antibiotics and preventive vaccines, it looked to many as if the ultimate victory against these microbial armies was imminent. Accompanying such delusions of victory has been a collective underestimation of the remarkable and highly unpredictable power of infection. As we see with each return of a seriously contagious epidemic, be it naturally induced or man-made, germs still have the ability to incite panic. Some have likened this relationship to a war between the species. I prefer to see it as an enduring dance among living beings in which the leading partner often changes with the passage of time. But the interactions of microbes and human beings demand far more than precise language to describe them. We require a different strategy for how we approach *all* health problems facing the world today.

Over the past century, sophisticated means of international public health surveillance and disease control have developed through experience, trial, and error. Nevertheless, these programs are expensive and tend to be underfunded because, paradoxically, public health and preventive medicine measures are silent by definition: if they are working well, few outbreaks of disease occur and those that do are contained quickly. This success, in turn, engenders public apathy or overconfidence that the "pitiless war," so nicely articulated by Hans Zinsser in 1935, has been won rather than stayed temporarily. Today, too many of us discount the value of public health programs, and given the ease and pace of international travel, dangerous microbes stand a better chance of gaining dominance.

I have written six chronicles of epidemics that span decades of medical progress as well as the two "great waves of immigration" to the United States. The first wave occurred from 1880 through 1924, when federal legislation closed the gates to newcomers for almost forty-one years because of native-born American fears that these people would change the social, political, economic, and even genetic face of the nation. The second wave of immigration began in 1965 and continues, in some fashion, to the present. During both of these periods, as many as a million immigrants arrived annually, not counting the undocumented or the foreign-born who simply visit. At present, more legal immigrants enter the United States each year than all of the other countries of the world combined, and our percentage of foreign-born citizens is the highest it has been since the 1920s.

Immigration in the twenty-first century is characterized by porous borders, rapid travel, and scattered destinations. While more than 75 percent of all immigrants during the first great wave of immigration came through New York harbor, immigrants today land at all the major airports across the United States with easy connections to cities and towns that do not have international arrivals. Moreover, jet transportation allows anyone to travel to the United States from the farthest reaches of the globe, giving public health physicians little opportunity to definitively diagnose infectious diseases silently incubating in a particular traveler. Although we currently possess a huge medical armamentarium, by the time an infectious disease becomes obvious the potentially ill immigrant is likely to have long since left the point of entry, making the spread of epidemics far more than a theoretical concern.

While most of us remain firmly convinced that the tradition of welcoming newcomers constitutes one of the finest variables of the American experiment, we cannot deny or ignore the risks of imported infection. In recent years, these perils have been magnified by human migration or settlement in areas not previously inhabited by humans and rising rates of deadly infectious diseases around the world. At the same time, we have witnessed rising numbers of illegal and undocumented immigrants entering the country who are unlikely to seek medical care for fear of legal repercussions and financial reasons. Equally grave, our nation's response to these problems has often been the allocation of fewer economic resources to maintain adequate disease control, and many legislators and policymakers have urged restricting access to health care for all aliens residing in the United States.

Underpinning these trends is a failure to embrace the unsettling fact that in the twenty-first century, the global village is host to a burgeoning community of dangerous and contagious microbes, some that kill relatively few in spectacular fashion, such as Ebola virus and SARS, and others such as tuberculosis that each year quietly, relentlessly, take the lives of millions. These pathogens demand far more respect and action than mere attempts at isolation or foolhardy efforts to build a wall around our nation.

This danger is not always apparent, however. Years ago I calculated the percentage of immigrants prevented from entering the United States between 1892 and 1924 because of a medical reason of any kind (including psychiatric and chronic as well as contagious diseases). It was miniscule, about one percent of the millions who sought entry each year. In fact, the most common reasons for the exclusion of immigrants during this period were abject poverty (officially, "Likely to Become a Public Charge"), followed by evidence that the immigrant was a criminal, a contract laborer, or a member of the "immoral classes" (that is, a prostitute).

One afternoon I proudly cited these statistics to the late immigration historian and social critic Irving Howe. He brusquely waved me away, much as my Yiddish-speaking grandfather would tell me to *Gay aveck!* (go away) when I bothered him with an impertinent question or comment. "It doesn't matter. It doesn't matter at all," he intoned, "because everyone knew someone—or someone who knew someone who was sent back because of a terrible disease. Every immigrant feared that an American doctor would suddenly pronounce them as ill or a danger to others even if they felt completely fine." Of course, Professor Howe was right. In the diaries and memoirs of immigrants arriving during the early twentieth century, one repeatedly encounters evidence of the intense fear of the physicians at Ellis Island, the medical inspection process, and the potential for deportation. Matters between the American doctor and the immigrant patient were rarely improved once the immigrant settled into his or her new home. Many avoided physicians entirely. Others lived in squalid conditions or may have adopted behaviors and habits that put them at high risk for developing diseases. Sadly, the relationship between many American doctors and immigrant patients continues to be characterized by this sense of uneasiness and, at times, outright avoidance.

Medical historians often study how responses to disease are socially constructed or shaped by nonbiological factors. We attempt to gather as much data as possible about a particular era's social institutions, cultural perceptions, daily activities, and other variables to re-create a complete sense of the past. But such an approach often overlooks the patient's actual experience with illness. Disease is socially constructed until you happen to find yourself in bed with one. On the other hand, physicians conduct diagnostic inquiries on a far more socially microscopic level. The longer I've practiced the craft of historical inquiry, the more I've grown to appreciate the medical diagnostician's approach to taking a history and trying to piece together different parts of a patient's life, experiences, and encounters with illness. This book represents an attempt to bring together the practices of medicine and medical history.

William Carlos Williams, a pediatrician who for almost fifty years maintained a busy practice in his own clinic, in the Paterson school district, and at the Passaic General Hospital in New Jersey, often wrote his poems and stories in between seeing patients or at the end of the day. While he is remembered for poems such as "The Red Wheelbarrow" and "Asphodel, That Greeny Flower," his short stories and essays include some of the most penetrating explorations of illness ever written.

Toward the end of his life, Dr. Williams described how his years of clinical encounters with patients allowed him a glimpse into the "underground stream" of humanity. "It is then we see, by this constant feeling

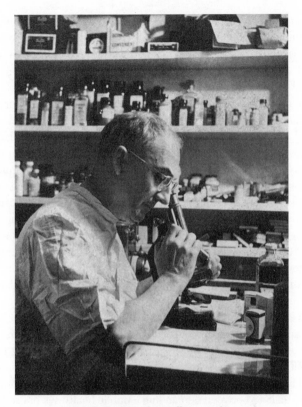

*Dr. William Carlos Williams in his*
*clinical laboratory, circa 1951*

for a meaning, from the unselected nature of the material, just as it comes in over the phone or at the office door, that there is no better way to get an intimation of what is going on in the world."[7]

There is, after all, something extraordinary about the transaction that takes place in a tiny clinic room occupied only by a physician and a person seeking a medical consultation. What is so surprising, especially to young doctors and not a few laypeople, is how often these talks have very little to do with the diseases and symptoms one finds neatly described in a medical textbook. Even in our era of wonder drugs, technological marvels that allow us to peer into the deepest recesses of the body, and awe-inspiring cures, skilled physicians place a high premium on the acts of observing patients and listening to their "histories"—what brought them to the clinic or hospital in the first place. Dr. Williams reminded us that this interaction not only allows the physician and patient to gain "a peace of mind" about a particular problem; they can also begin "to build a reasonable basis for action which really gives us our peace."[8]

As he contemplated the threads common to the crafts of storytelling, poetry, history, and doctoring, Dr. Williams concluded, "The poet's business [is] not to talk in vague categories but to write particularly, as a physician works, upon a patient, upon the thing before him, in the particular to discover the universal."[9] This is the charge that has guided me in writing these doctor's stories of imported infection. They include traditional historical accounts as well as contemporary tales that are more akin to personal memoir. Some are drawn from archives dating back to the first great wave of American immigration. A few describe the experiences of those who were either my own or my colleagues' patients. Each is an attempt to understand the world of many living beings: immigrants, physicians, concerned observers, patients, and, of course, the dangerous germs they encountered.

I have chosen these particular American stories because I am an American historian and practice medicine in the United States. But I hope that they illustrate universal truths about the enduring relationships between microbes and human beings and between the sick and those charged with protecting the well. Taken together, the stories show how we vacillate between demanding a public health system so punitive that it worsens matters rather than protects, and settling for one that is too lax; and between being fascinated with all things infectious to hardly giving microbes a second thought.

# ONE

## Facing Tuberculosis

For me, the awful—almost physically painful—loneliness began the minute I heard a young doctor utter the phrase "TB" as an explanation for my problems. Two letters! Who would have thought that someone articulating so brief a phrase would have so much power to completely change your life?

— ABDUL, an Ethiopian immigrant, reflecting
on his initial diagnosis of tuberculosis[1]

One afternoon a month and a day after the terrorist attacks on the World Trade Center and the Pentagon, I was in a crowded subway car making its way down Manhattan's Upper West Side. Only seven miles south of the 125th Street station, where the train was delayed temporarily, rescue workers and firemen were searching through the rubble and carnage of September 11, 2001. Yet on the subway that afternoon—and around the country—a different form of terror was on our minds.

Directly above me on both sides of the train were bright posters advertising a new and improved detergent that "eliminates 99.9% of all bacteria lurking in your clothing." (Parenthetically, all soaps pretty much accomplish this task.) Sitting next to me was a heavyset woman rubbing her hands over and over like some modern-day Lady Macbeth. Only instead of washing off the blood of her royal rivals, she was slathering her hands with a pinkish red anti-bacterial moisturizer "guaranteed to both soften the skin and rid you of nasty germs." Seated next to her were two older men who appeared to be breathing less deeply and far more rapidly than I suspected they might otherwise be doing. At the very end of the car was a young woman wearing a surgical mask and rubber gloves.

If these signs were not enough to alert the casual observer to what was going on, all one had to do was glance at the newspapers many were reading. Every publication, from the lowly tabloids to the august *New York Times*, screamed the same headline in bold print: ANTHRAX! Inside their pages were all the sordid details of the infection-laden letters sent earlier that week to Senator Tom Daschle and others. That very morning, an assistant to NBC anchorman Tom Brokaw, who received a similar missive in late September, was confirmed to have a bona fide case of cutaneous anthrax.

In the weeks that followed, several more cases of anthrax popped up, some easily explained (such as those among the postal workers handling the tainted mail) and some not (such as the fatal case in an elderly woman from Connecticut whose mail was, unluckily, mixed in with contaminated envelopes meant for others). And we all worried if the Pandora's box of germs that appeared to have been opened by terrorists would ever be closed. The sudden appearance of a frightening, infectious agent was, perhaps, one of the few things that could have so successfully taken the nation's collective mind, albeit temporarily, off the stunning events at ground zero. Government officials searched to find the source of the infection, to the accompaniment of television pundits pointing fingers and calling our public health mechanisms inadequate. Sales of Cipro, one of several antibiotics effective against anthrax (and by far the most expensive), went through the roof. Emergency rooms and clinics across the country were inundated with people wondering if every scrape, wheeze, or contact with something as harmless as the crumbs of a powdered sugar doughnut was an incipient case of anthrax.[2]

That the public would focus with a laser beam intensity on anthrax, a strange scourge that killed only a few in spectacular fashion, while paying little attention to the more common contagions that literally plague us on a daily basis, is a phenomenon hardly unique to our era. Healthy human beings frequently worry more about frightening, unexpected infections than about diseases we know all too well, such as tuberculosis, a disease that is slow and patient, relentless and effective, and year in, year out, sends millions to their graves.[3] If the forces of evolutionary biology could have imbued the tuberculosis germ with the capacity to feel neglect, it was probably used to it by now.

Today, more than 2 billion of the planet's 6 billion people are infected with the latent form of tuberculosis. In the United States alone, 10 to 15 million are infected with it. Of this multitude, at least 10 percent of them will go on to develop the active form of tuberculosis sometime during their lives. The period between latency (with no signs of disease at all except a positive TB skin test) and active illness can range from weeks to years after the microbe *Mycobacterium tuberculosis* settles into the human body. Much has to do with the health of the particular host, his nutritional status, living conditions, and the coexistence of other dis-

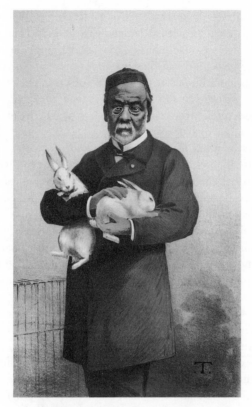

*The French chemist Louis Pasteur
(1822–1895) theorized in the 1860s that
microbes, or "germs," were the cause of
infectious or contagious diseases.*

eases. But when considering the many influences that enable the TB
bacillus to transform good health to ill, it is wise to recall the French
chemist and microbiologist Louis Pasteur's warning to respect the "infinitely great power of the infinitely small."[4]

Every year public health officials across the globe diagnose more than
8 million active cases of TB. These are the people who are most infectious to others. The sicker someone is with active TB, the greater the
number of microbes in his or her body; and with every cough, shout, or
breath, that individual becomes a more significant risk to the public

health. The average person with active TB will infect twenty other people before he or she dies or is adequately treated. What surprises many is that during every twelve-month period, about 3 million people die of tuberculosis, making it the leading infectious cause of death in the world today. In fact, more human beings will die of TB in our era than at any other point in recorded history.

The disease, often referred to as the white plague in deference to the infamous bubonic, or black plague, typically strikes adults during their most productive years of life, ages eighteen to fifty-five. Fortunately, since the late 1940s medicine has been blessed with a wide range of potent antibiotics that can treat TB and, in most cases, cure it. At the same time, these medical miracles have given rise to premature declarations of victory over tuberculosis. Especially over the past decade, public health specialists have grown concerned about the rise of multidrug-resistant strains of tuberculosis around the world. In layman's terms, this means that not only do we have deadly germs on our hands, but, in at least one out of ten cases (and far more in Asia, South America, and the former Soviet Union), the mycobacteria are resistant to the very menu of powerful drugs we have developed to enter and kill them.

Only recently have we begun to recognize the folly of extensive funding cuts in tuberculosis surveillance and treatment programs, and the unintended consequences of not investing in the basic health care needs of the most impoverished citizens of the world. Moreover, with the rise of HIV/AIDS over the past two decades, there is now a significant population of immunocompromised individuals who are highly susceptible to TB and can potentially spread the disease like an uncontrollable wildfire. Major social upheavals during these years have also resulted in mass migration movements around the globe. Each of these factors has created the conditions the tubercle bacillus needs to thrive once again, inspiring the World Health Organization to classify tuberculosis as "a global health emergency."[5] My fellow subway passengers that afternoon may have been worried about the off chance of meeting an anthrax spore. A few may have been contemplating the risk of a terrorist delivery of smallpox virus or even the highly unlikely importation of Ebola virus. I was, and am, far more concerned about contracting TB.

Few stories of tuberculosis demonstrate its unpredictability better than that of one of the immigrants I met in a professor's office near the New York–Presbyterian Hospital Tuberculosis Clinic. Alejandro, a fifty-year-old laborer who came to the United States illegally from Ecuador in 1999, was a relatively new patient at the clinic and had just been declared "noncontagious" after a four-week hospital stay.[6] In Quito, he had been employed as a building contractor's assistant and "worked twelve or more hours a day, six to seven days a week, for over twenty-nine years." As with many immigrants before and since, economic insecurity was his major impetus for leaving Ecuador: "The price of food in Quito—the price of everything—is very high. We simply could not make it in my country. So I decided I had to go to America alone, whatever the cost, to bring in more money for my family."

In the late summer of 1999, Alejandro left his wife and three sons to begin a dangerous and illegal trip to the United States. The trip actually began months before when he procured the services of a coyote, a nefarious "travel agent" who specializes in smuggling human cargo across international borders. Alejandro met the coyote through some friends in Quito, although he noted that these "professionals" advertise in newspapers and are relatively easy to find. Alejandro's coyote was "a well-dressed, slick guy who promised a safe journey using his extensive network of contacts, the best means of travel, good food, everything." But the "travel package" came at a steep price: $7,000. This sum, several times more than Alejandro's annual income, required him to take out a mortgage on his family home. However, the financial transaction was not executed at a bank. The entire deal, even down to a payment plan that charged 5 percent interest per month, was completed between the two men on the street in front of Alejandro's house. Each month since he signed the paperwork for this deal, Alejandro has wired the coyote $250.

From Ecuador, without passport, visa, or luggage, Alejandro flew in a tiny propeller plane to the desert in southern Mexico. He then traveled across the interior toward Ciudad Juárez over a four-day period. For this leg of the journey, his means of transportation was the back of a dilapidated pickup truck squeezed in between forty-nine other illegal immigrants. To avoid the Mexican authorities, they drove a circuitous route along bumpy back roads. Alejandro rubbed his rear end as he recalled this part of his trip and remarked, "I can still feel every rock and pothole." Each night they slept outside and were sold a ration of food. A plate of rice and beans, Alejandro recalled, cost "about ten dollars."

Once the truck reached Ciudad Juárez, it was simply a matter of crossing the Rio Grande into El Paso. But the U.S. immigration workers stopped the truck as soon as it attempted to pass the border, and the briefest of inspections justified their suspicions. All fifty illegal immigrants—Ecuadorans, Nicaraguans, Panamanians, and a few Mexicans—were taken to jail. Following their instructions from the coyote, each immigrant told the Immigration and Naturalization Service (INS) officers they were seeking political asylum.

Alejandro sat in an El Paso jail for almost six weeks, but recalled it as a far better living arrangement than what he had endured during his travels. He was brought before the immigration court and required to post a $3,000 bail bond. Fortunately, he was able to contact some relatives who had long ago settled in New York, and they wired this princely sum to the authorities. The judge questioned Alejandro through an interpreter and allowed him to be released provided he return for a more definitive hearing at a later date. Naturally, Alejandro agreed to these terms and promptly gave the bailiff a fictional address at which to contact him. Soon after, he assumed a false name and purchased a bus ticket to New York. He had no papers, no legal identity, not even claim to his given name. He was an undocumented immigrant. His is hardly an exceptional tale. At present, while two-thirds of the illegal immigrants arrested along the Mexican and Canadian borders voluntarily return to their lands of origin, of those who remain, 90 percent never show up for their hearings, and little if any effort is made to find them.[7]

A few weeks after Alejandro arrived in New York City, he found a job at a delicatessen in the downtown financial district. Alejandro's physician told me later that about half of the illegal immigrants in New York work in the food services industry. To be sure, those with active tuberculosis do not pose the same immediate health risks to unsuspecting diners as "Typhoid Mary" Mallon, the cook who caused several *Salmonella* outbreaks in New York City during the early twentieth century.[8] Nevertheless, the possibility that an illegal immigrant harboring a contagious disease with little or no access to health care is preparing your next egg salad sandwich, at the very least, should seriously curb your appetite.

At the deli, Alejandro worked fourteen hours a day, six days a week performing tasks such as cleaning up the tables, making sandwiches, and restocking the bountiful salad bar that nourished the harried stockbrokers, lawyers, and office workers who came in for a quick meal. He was paid about $500 a week, always in cash. After covering his own room and board and the coyote's monthly fee, whatever money he had left over each month Alejandro wired to his wife in Ecuador.

Despite these hardships Alejandro observed, "Everything was working out fine until this past summer." At that point, the tubercle bacilli he may have inhaled in Ecuador or even in the United States activated with a vengeance, causing intense sweating, fatigue, and difficulty standing upright. "At first, I blamed it on the hard work," Alejandro explained, "the long hours, the summer heat. But these problems would not go away. No matter how much rest I got on Sundays, I still felt terrible. Worse than I ever felt in my entire life. I had these headaches, terrible, it felt like someone was hitting me over the head with a brick."

Alejandro lived in a small two-room apartment with eight other Ecuadoran men, all illegal immigrants, on the Harlem side of Morningside Park, just a few blocks from Columbia University. They fashioned cardboard partitions between their beds to give some sense of privacy, but there was little to be had. Victor, a middle-aged man who slept in the bed next to Alejandro and worked with him at the delicatessen downtown, insisted that he see a doctor. One Monday morning, the two men skipped work and made a visit to a Spanish-speaking physician on West Ninety-sixth Street. Alejandro later complained: "He didn't ask me to take my shirt off. He didn't take any blood, get an X-ray, nothing." Instead, the physician stopped his inquiry after hearing the words "terrible headaches" and prescribed a new anti-inflammatory pain reliever named Vioxx. The pills did little for Alejandro's headaches, but their $70 price tag plus the doctor's $50 fee wreaked havoc on his carefully calibrated budget.

By early September, disgusted by the Latino doctor and still troubled by his worsening headaches and exhaustion, Alejandro decided to go to the New York–Presbyterian Hospital's emergency room for medical advice. Soon after he arrived, the triage nurse deemed Alejandro too well for evaluation in the ER and he was escorted across the street to the Urgent Care Clinic. There, at least, a nurse took his blood pressure and listened to his chest, but the examination went no further. Alejandro was sent on his way with another prescription for Vioxx.

During the second week of September 2001, Alejandro was simply too ill to go to work. On September 10, Victor took his ailing friend to still another doctor who also catered to a Spanish-speaking immigrant clientele. That afternoon their angry boss sent word that they were both fired. Finally, on September 16, the pounding headaches, an inability to walk, and incoherent speech led Victor to call an ambulance to rush Alejandro back to the New York–Presbyterian Hospital. An X-ray of his chest revealed extensive cavitary disease (in other words, a large hole) in his right lung. Worse still, a spinal tap to extract a sample of cerebrospinal fluid that bathes the brain demonstrated that the mycobacteria had invaded Alejandro's central nervous system. He now had an excellent explanation for his terrible headaches and dizziness: tuberculosis meningitis.

As he sat across from me one month later, I would never have guessed that this large muscular man was so recently close to death. But while Alejandro was now on the road to recovery, his doctors remained concerned about the people he came in close contact with, such as his roommates. None of them had yet been tested for tuberculosis because the appointments they were given were all during working hours, Monday through Friday. "My friends might lose their jobs, like I did, if they did the right thing and get tested," Alejandro explained. "They leave for work at seven in the morning and come home at ten at night. Maybe things would be better for everyone if the doctors had Sunday hours or came to our neighborhood. My friends could get tested and treated, and maybe the infections would stop." As with many illegal immigrants, on further inquiry Alejandro admitted that he and most of his friends studiously avoided American doctors out of fear of legal repercussions and deportation.[9]

Alejandro insisted that neither his health nor his legal problems weighed as heavily on his mind as did his financial instability and its impact on his family. At the close of our meeting, I asked him exactly where the delicatessen he was fired from on September 10 was located. He quickly replied, "Right across the street from the World Trade Center." With a smile and a shrug, Alejandro added, "You know, if it were not for my having tuberculosis, I might have been dead today."

The rapid international travel of people harboring deadly germs represents a real public health challenge. A thirty-two-year-old South Korean woman whose bout with tuberculosis made national headlines in 1996 was treated several times for tuberculosis (twice as a teenager and a third time in 1992), and her doctors gave her a clean bill of health. She was taking no medication in February 1994 when she applied for a tourist's visa to the United States, and shortly thereafter, in early March, Soon-Ye boarded a plane from Seoul, South Korea, to Honolulu. During this period, obtaining a tourist visa was a relatively simple matter that required no medical examination, let alone a TB screening test. Much is made about the roughly one million immigrants who come to the United

States each year to settle. More concern is typically paid to the 250,000 to 500,000 illegal aliens who also arrive annually. But it is important to recall that especially in the years before post-9/11 travel security measures, some 50 million foreign travelers visited the United States each year as well, few of whom underwent any type of medical scrutiny.

Soon-Ye stayed in Honolulu for five days. Her hosts later reported that she was coughing a lot and appeared tired. At the time, however, these symptoms were ascribed to her arduous journey. After a brief stopover at Chicago's O'Hare Airport, Soon-Ye flew to Baltimore, where she stayed at the home of another set of friends for about a month.

Within a few days there, her symptoms worsened. Soon-Ye's cough was now so loud and persistent that it kept the entire household awake at night. She complained of raging fevers and nightly bouts of intense sweating. Worse was the extreme fatigue that made even a trip to the bathroom an almost insurmountable task. Perhaps the most specific sign of Soon-Ye's deathly illness was her coughing up blood—a symptom physicians refer to as hemoptysis and an effective pathological announcement that the tuberculosis germs had destroyed enough lung tissue to invade the rich bed of arterioles and arteries surrounding them. Throughout the ordeal, Soon-Ye rarely complained or talked much about the havoc going on deep inside her chest. One of her friends later explained that Soon-Ye's stoicism was a common response to serious disease among Korean women.

In early May, Soon-Ye flew back to Honolulu with the intention of returning to Seoul, but her hemoptysis would not stop. One fellow passenger later recalled with alarm that Soon-Ye went through dozens of handkerchiefs during the flight, each of them rapidly turned from a snowy white to a bright red. In terms of the spread of tuberculosis, there is probably no stage more contagious. After one day in Hawaii, her friends took her to a hospital where X-rays revealed extensive damage of her lungs. That very afternoon she coughed up more than a liter of blood. Within a few days, bacterial cultures and DNA analyses of the bloody ooze originating from her decimated lungs were overwhelmingly positive for a multidrug-resistant strain of *Mycobacterium tuberculosis*. Her doctors were unable to stop the bleeding, and despite their valiant efforts she was dead before the week was over.

In the months that followed, a team of physicians and epidemiologists tracked down 925 (88.8%) of the 1,042 passengers who traveled with Soon-Ye on these four flights. After excluding 40 passengers who were already known to be infected with latent tuberculosis and 2 others who died of AIDS and cancer shortly after the flights, the microbe hunters tested the remaining passengers for TB exposure. Seven passengers on flight one (Seoul to Honolulu) were positive, 4 on flight two (Honolulu to Chicago), 3 on flight three (Chicago to Baltimore), and 15 on flight four (Baltimore to Honolulu). Based on the epidemiological evidence at hand, the worst-case scenario suggested Soon-Ye infected 29 other people on these flights alone. The riskiest place to sit, not surprisingly, was within a few rows of her.

Although short flights (those less than eight hours) and air filtration systems on jetliners today tend to protect the overwhelming majority of air travelers from contracting tuberculosis on a plane containing contagious passengers, Soon-Ye's story demonstrates how air travel can pose a risk to one's health. Indeed, since 1996 all the world's major public health organizations have worried about the transmission of TB during long transoceanic flights, especially those originating from regions in the world where it is endemic.[10]

Tuberculosis is an easily acquired infection, provided a susceptible person spends significant time breathing the same air as another who is actively suffering from the disease. Each time someone with tuberculosis coughs, sneezes, or even yells or sings, he expels droplets of saliva, phlegm, and tuberculosis bacilli into the air. Physicists have even worked out mathematical formulas to describe the arc and speed of these droplets as they take off from the mouth. Coughing turns out to be one of the most efficient means of spreading respiratory infections, and those of us who used to ignore our mother's warnings to breathe gingerly around people with a cough should reconsider this sagacious advice.[11]

Every day human beings inhale huge numbers of dangerous particles, be they germs, dust, or environmental toxins. Fortunately, long before these substances get into the lungs where they can do the most damage, they must traverse a long and winding road of air passages—the trachea, bronchi, and bronchioles. Along the sides of these pulmonary byways are goblet cells that secrete droplets of sticky mucus which trap most of the offensive invaders. As an added protection, these cells are equipped with cilia, tiny hairs that move in waves, much like an escalator that only goes up, to expel the foreigners as far away from the lungs as possible. One of the many unhealthy side effects of cigarette smoking, incidentally, is that the hot smoke paralyzes these cilia and essentially stops their up-escalator motion, making smokers more at risk for all kinds of respiratory infections. For most of us, however, the denouement to these scenes of entrapment is a robust and, at times, messy cough.[12]

In terms of spreading infection, the size of the particles coughed up by someone with tuberculosis is critical. Large droplets of saliva succumb to the forces of gravity and tend to settle quickly to the ground or the nearest surface. But smaller saliva droplets and even tinier germs can actually float about for several hours with the sole ambition of being inhaled by another warm body. To help make this point clearer, let's consider some metric perspectives. One of the smallest living beings visible to the naked eye is a human egg cell. This basic entity of life is about 100 microns in width. A human hair, while long in length, is only about 75 microns in width. A human skin cell is small enough to be invisible to the naked eye, about 10 microns in width. But bacteria, mycobacteria, and viruses are far more troublesome to prospective patients and their doctors because they are often less than 2 microns in diameter and are among the world's smallest independent living beings. It is precisely these microbes that are the most adept at floating in the air and, when inhaled by others, passing through the airways.[13] Such intrepid travelers often avoid both the sticky mucous traps and the wavy cilia. They then make their way into the alveoli, the tiny air sacs of the lungs where the real work of respiration takes place: inhaled and life-giving oxygen molecules are exchanged into the bloodstream for the waste product we know (and exhale) as carbon dioxide.

It is in the alveoli where the infection of tuberculosis essentially begins. Resident in these lithe, membranous air bubbles are immune cells, front-line soldiers really, called macrophages. Unlike many other cells that play prominent roles in the human immune system's version of Armageddon that takes place countless times a day, macrophages are neither elegant nor intellectually appealing. They are the immunological equivalent of garbagemen. These mobile cells patrol a given area and remove the foreign particles and damaged cellular debris the body has cast aside. Their collections run the gamut from a tiny piece of ash you may inhale because your next-door neighbor is burning leaves all the way to deadly microbes.

The problem most of us have with the tuberculosis germ is that it is remarkably adept at resisting our body's attempt to destroy it. Despite the macrophage's ability to swallow the germ whole and the battery of harsh chemical agents it carries in its physiological backpack, the mycobacterium's thick, waxy coating is often quite good at protecting itself from final annihilation. As a result of TB's armor, the bloated macrophage cannot always digest the entire meal it has taken. The surviving mycobacteria subsequently live and multiply in the macrophage while patiently plotting the next battle, be it in the lungs themselves (the favorite spot), lymph nodes, or off into the bloodstream to find another fertile Gettysburg.[14]

*Mycobacterium tuberculosis* makes its primary home in the lungs for a good reason: it is an organism that requires great concentrations of oxygen to thrive. Consequently, TB germs prefer the apex, or tip, of the lung because it is that portion of our breathing apparatus that is most rich in oxygen. Readers of Thomas Mann's novel *The Magic Mountain* will recall that the sanatorium where the hero, Hans Castorp, is sent is situated high in the Alps.[15] The location of many, though certainly not all, tuberculosis sanatoria in high altitudes was a serendipitous and therapeutic discovery. During the second half of the nineteenth century, long before anything was specifically known about the germ of tuberculosis, physicians observed that TB patients recuperated faster in areas where the oxygen content of the air was thin, hence the "Magic Mountain." These doctors also concluded that the accompanying cold weather was curative, and as a result, generations of TB patients were forced to sleep outside in cold, snowy locales. This latter therapeutic measure, however, probably benefited only the manufacturers of winter coats and heavy woolen blankets.[16]

After the mycobacterium settles into the lungs of a victim, it can inspire an aggressive primary infection or it can quiet itself and reside there for months to years before reactivating. When the stalemate between the germ's offensive line and the host's immune defenses tips in favor of the germ, the real war begins. At this point, the multiplying mycobacteria destroy more and more of the lung as they form tubercles, the mass of microbes, macrophages, and other spent immune cells clustered around a core of dead, rotting tissue that pathologists quaintly refer to as caseous (from the Latin for "cheeselike") necrosis. Initially, a patient may simply complain of a dry, hacking cough. But as the disease progresses and the infected person's immune system mounts an all-out effort to fight off these invaders, one experiences raging bouts of fever, drenching sweats, typically at night, and utter exhaustion.

During the 1920s, physicians tried to outsmart the TB germ's voracious appetite for oxygen and developed a surgical procedure called pneumothorax. It causes the collapse of a tubercular lung by placing a hole in the side of the chest. By minimizing the oxygen content of a diseased lung and giving it a rest, surgeons hoped to starve the tuberculosis infection to death. In some cases this method worked, and in many more others it did not. Up to the 1960s, surgeons routinely removed part or all of a diseased lung in a desperate attempt to cure the most stubborn cases. Unfortunately, with the advent of drug-resistant cases of tuberculosis, this gruesome, but at times lifesaving, procedure has made a comeback.[17]

Although tuberculosis is primarily a disease of the lungs, once it enters the lymphatic system or catches a ride into the bloodstream, it can set up shop in almost any part of the susceptible body. Sometimes the mycobacteria commandeer the cervical lymph nodes near the surface of the skin of the neck, a condition doctors have long called scrofula. The infected lymph glands transform into knotted masses, inflame the skin, and, worse, break through to the surface, leaving an unsightly river of pus on the back or underside of one's neck. Among the most illustrious scrofula sufferers was the legendary British literary critic Samuel Johnson.[18] Other times, the microbe can settle in the larynx or voice box, which makes the very act of speaking a contagious event and ultimately silences its victim; and when the germs are swallowed, they can multiply in the intestines, where they cause a painful and relentless diarrhea.

More threatening, mycobacteria can attack the kidneys, transforming these critical blood filters and urine factories into clogged, useless hunks of dead tissue. Or they can detonate in the bones. The spinal column is a particularly favored spot, and the tuberculosis germs can erode this essential scaffolding so it ultimately collapses upon itself. This bony destruction is called Pott's disease, after the eighteenth-century British surgeon Percival Pott who first described it. One of the most painful conclusions of TB, however, occurs when it invades and destroys the brain, a condition called tuberculosis meningitis.

The ancient Greeks had a word to describe the disease's ravages: *phthisis,* related to the root *phthoe,* which describes a living body that shrivels with intense heat as if placed on a flame. Later, the Romans applied the Latin word *consumere,* to eat up or devour, to the malady.[19] Well into the twentieth century, when it was one of the leading causes of death in the United States, many Americans still referred to tuberculosis as consumption. This is precisely what active TB does. It consumes with a passionate and incisive energy, slowly, inexorably devouring the very structure of the lungs and other critical organs with the single goal of conquering its host; but not until its progeny have had the opportunity to travel to the lungs of another human being in order to start the horrific process all over again.

Much has been written about the romantic nature of tuberculosis. It is, after all, the disease that carried away the poet John Keats and the Brontë sisters; the illness that likely rang down the final curtain on the lives of Molière, Voltaire, and Chekhov. Mention the word "tuberculosis" and many music lovers can almost visualize Frédéric Chopin trying to compose a nocturne while violently coughing at the keyboard. The powerful closing scenes of Verdi's *La Traviata* and Puccini's *La Bohème* both feature beautiful heroines struck down by TB. As a result, several scholars have characterized tuberculosis as the perfect operatic disease, a mysterious entity that robs one of breath, voice, and ultimately life. Opera buffs are not alone in extolling the charms of the white plague. The novelist and literary critic Susan Sontag describes the malady in her book *Illness as Metaphor* as "an aphrodisiac," a disease with "extraordinary power of seduction."[20]

When seated in a plush opera house watching the beautiful alabaster-pale Violetta collapse to the stirring orchestral themes of *Traviata,* who can help being enchanted and seduced by the power of tuberculosis? In real life, the illness is a messy, agonizing, and debilitating ordeal. Latent tuberculosis tends not to inspire obvious symptoms, although its mere diagnosis may be subtly exotic for some. But once the tubercle bacilli gain the momentum to proceed unchecked through the body, there is little romance to be found. The experience of active tuberculosis is one of exhaustion, not literary inspiration; drenching bouts of sweating, not hypersexual allure; irritable groaning, not lyrical arias; a relentless cough punctuated with spurts of blood, not the lover's kiss. This is the nightmarish reality of the white plague.

In many respects, the modern era of tuberculosis began in the mind of a twenty-nine-year-old German physician named Robert Koch, who in 1872 was appointed the district medical officer in Wollstein (a tiny village in West Prussia, now Wolsztyn, Poland). The Koch family lived in a four-room wooden-frame home, and the doctor's consulting area was situated in the house's parlor. Using a simple curtain to divide this room in half, Koch set up a laboratory that consisted of nothing more than a

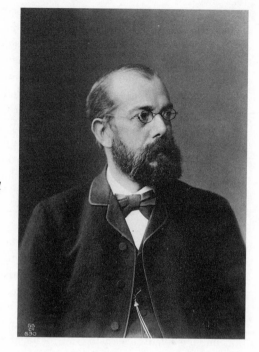

*The German physician Robert Koch (1843–1910) discovered the germs that cause anthrax, cholera, and tuberculosis.*

microscope he had specially ordered from Berlin, an incubator, sundry glass tubes, culture plates and retorts, and a camera he had rigged to the microscope to photograph microbes.[21]

Like many young physicians of this era, Koch was stricken by an intense fascination with all things microscopic, a fixation some medical critics derided as "bacteriomania."[22] Unlike his senior colleagues who ascribed epidemics to the contamination of the air with foul or unpleasant emanations (the miasmatic theory), Koch sided with those who would become the scientific revolutionaries of their day by asserting and ultimately proving that specific germs were the seat of the cause of illnesses like cholera, diphtheria, and bubonic plague.

Because Dr. Koch practiced in an agricultural district where wool production was a major industry, he saw his share of anthrax patients. Most of the cases he treated were what we call today cutaneous anthrax, a painful coal black (hence, the name anthrax, from anthracite) sore on the fingers or hands that results from physical contact with the microbes. But in the most severe situations, what we now refer to as inhalational anthrax, the germs entered the lungs of unsuspecting wool-gatherers who soon enough succumbed to raging fevers, hemorrhaging, and death. Like many physicians, Koch believed that these workers were somehow ingesting a microscopic organism living on the hides of animal carcasses, but his knowledge ended there. Helpless at his patients' bedside, Koch was determined to figure out anthrax's cause and, if possible, find a cure. So every evening, after the last patient had left his consulting room, the young physician retired behind his curtain, sat at his makeshift laboratory bench, peered through the barrel of his microscope, and conducted his search. Within a few months after he began this work, and countless mice later, Koch had his answer. A microbe named *Bacillus anthracis,* he painstakingly determined, caused anthrax.

Serendipity can be one of the most important components of a scientific discovery, yet as Louis Pasteur liked to quip, "chance favors only the prepared mind."[23] Three physical characteristics of *Bacillus anthracis* favored Koch's discovery. The microbe has a distinctive appearance under a microscope, it is a large germ that forms even larger and very hardy spores that can survive almost any manner of physical manipulation, and it is relatively easy to grow in the laboratory.

In the spring of 1876, Koch traveled seventy-five miles south to Breslau (now Wroclaw, Poland) to meet the celebrated botanist and bacteriologist Ferdinand Cohn. At Cohn's well-equipped laboratory, Koch presented his research findings on anthrax. Cohn repeated the experiments and, with great joy, personally put his considerable stamp of approval on the country doctor's nocturnal tinkering by arranging to have Koch's seminal work published.

Despite his remarkable achievement of being the first person to scientifically link a specific germ to a specific disease and the ringing endorsements of a number of illustrious professors across Europe, Koch was unable to find a university position that allowed him the time and facilities to pursue his research full-time. And so he remained in Wollstein for another four years, until 1880, when he was appointed government advisor to the Imperial Department of Health in Berlin.

It was there that Koch began a series of pathbreaking discoveries that led to his winning the Nobel Prize for medicine or physiology in 1905. With a superb laboratory, powerful microscopes, and all the assistants, experimental animals, and materials he could ask for, Koch decided to investigate one of the major killers of his day: tuberculosis. His research focus was quite controversial at the time because most experts insisted that TB was a hereditary disease; after all, it *did* tend to run in families. Nevertheless, Dr. Koch was convinced that TB was infectious in nature. Working alone, without telling his colleagues, he locked himself in his laboratory every day for almost six months until he definitively isolated the germ that we now know causes the disease: the tubercle bacillus, or *Mycobacterium tuberculosis.*

Never a commanding lecturer, Koch had a thin, reedy voice and tended to interject his phrases with an annoying amount of "ums" and "ers." But on March 24, 1882, when he presented his findings before the Physiological Society of Berlin, he did so with clarity and elegant logic, and the audience of doctors and scientists was dumbstruck. So spellbound and conscious of the fact that they were witnesses to scientific history, they could not even applaud, let alone engage in the traditional doctorly attack on another colleague's work. In the auditorium was a young dermatologist named Paul Ehrlich, who ultimately achieved great fame as the discoverer of Salvarsan 606, the first "magic bullet" against syphilis. Ehrlich later recalled the evening as "the most gripping experience" of his scientific life, and as soon as the lecture was completed he went home to his makeshift laboratory, where he spent the night developing a novel staining technique for the tubercle bacillus.[24]

In the decades that followed, physicians and public health experts around the world rushed to develop the means to control and prevent the white plague. Long before antibiotics, the major strategy was a widescale educational campaign to teach the public how to both avoid tuberculosis and recognize its symptoms. Newspapers and magazines, posters, advertisements, pamphlets, comic-book primers, and even best-selling books on these topics were written in order to help promote good health.

Some of the most widely read books on tuberculosis in the United States during this era were written by the eminent physician, medical school professor, and bacteriologist T. Mitchell Prudden.[25] Between 1889 and 1891, Dr. Prudden wrote three popular tomes explaining the latest exciting discoveries being made about infectious diseases and how to avoid, if not entirely conquer them.[26] Without hesitation or fear of overstatement, Prudden assured his readers in 1890 that the conquest of deadly infectious scourges was at hand: "we no longer grope after some mysterious, intangible thing, before which we must bow down or burn something as if it were some demon which we would exorcise."[27]

Around this time, many physicians agreed that the greatest source of tuberculosis bacilli was sputum, the sticky, disgusting phlegm humans cough up when their lungs are infected or irritated by foreign invaders. But from the 1890s well into the 1920s a tuberculosis patient's penchant for coughing or breathing in the presence of others was *not* considered the major means of contagion. Instead, the leading theory of the day held that the white plague was spread by inconsiderate tuberculosis sufferers spitting out their gelatinous, tenacious sputum wherever they so wished. Americans of this era were hardly shy about such acts. They coughed, sneezed, and spat with free abandon and, too often, showed little concern that their crude habits might be at the root of an epidemic.[28]

Anti-tuberculosis crusaders like Prudden stayed awake at night worrying about the multitude of consumptives walking about "who discharge the infectious materials coughed up from the lungs upon the pavements or floors." From the unseemly act of expectoration, it was only a brief time before such slimy slobbering dried up and took its place "among the rest of the floating dust of the air" when it was then inhaled by the unsuspecting healthy.[29] Dr. Prudden and his colleagues were determined to change such social practices, and cajoled and scolded Americans to swallow the sputum they coughed up rather than spitting it out.

Public health departments published circulars emblazoned with warnings like "Spitting is dangerous, indecent and against the law."[30] People with tuberculosis were persuaded to cough and spit into handkerchiefs saturated with strong disinfectants or specially made cardboard "sputum boxes." Drinking fountains were equipped with disposable paper cups to discourage people from leaning over and spitting into them. All these and more curbs to the American "expectorate prerogative" were employed to prevent those with tuberculosis, both native-born and immigrants, from spreading their infection to other Americans.[31] Occasionally today, an observant visitor to an aging subway station in New York City will spy an old board of health placard emblazoned with the prohibitive warning "No Spitting." Most of us gladly heed this order out of an aesthetic sensibility or at least good manners, without ever realizing that the rule was once considered an important weapon in the war against tuberculosis.

Aside from spitting, another means of transmission perceived to be a threat was the simple act of kissing.[32] Once a diagnosis of tuberculosis was made, that person was forbidden to engage in this intimate act of

*Beginning in the 1880s and lasting well into the 1940s, many considered kissing to be a major means of transmitting tuberculosis.*

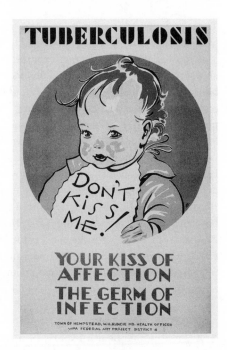

expression between lovers and loved ones. It is difficult to know how successful a no kissing edict was in arresting the spread of tuberculosis, although contemporary understanding of the disease suggests it is unlikely many cases were prevented by these doctor's orders. But the prohibitions, undoubtedly, helped to stigmatize and isolate those stricken with tuberculosis.

It was actually not until the 1960s that the airborne transmission of tuberculosis was scientifically demonstrated. In a six-bed ward at the Veterans Administration Hospital in Baltimore, a young physician named Richard Riley designed an ingenious way to prove a theory that his teacher at Harvard Medical School, Dr. William Wells, had been espousing since the 1930s. Riley assigned his TB patients to a special room, where they remained until their antibiotic treatment took hold and they were no longer considered contagious to others. What the patients did not know was that the ward was sealed in such a fashion that the air they expelled from their tubercular lungs was vented to a penthouse "exposure chamber" that housed hundreds of guinea pigs.

These rodents, whose name connotes the spirit of experimentation, are famously susceptible to *Mycobacterium tuberculosis.*

Almost all of the guinea pigs exposed to the tuberculosis-impregnated air soon contracted the illness. This fact was amply demonstrated by a beleaguered research assistant who had to perform hundreds of guinea pig autopsies in exchange for a sterling letter of recommendation to the medical school of his choosing. Subsequent analysis of the organisms isolated from the guinea pigs and comparisons to those from the human patients pretty much established the airborne transmission theory as fact. Later still, it was shown that in most cases, one must breathe in a lot of TB germs over a long period of time in order to contract the disease. But the exact period of time depends a great deal on the health status of both the person spreading the TB germs and the one inhaling them.[33] For example, those with the most extensive disease tend to be the most efficient carriers; and our ever-increasing experience with immunocompromised people with HIV or malignancies has demonstrated a whole new population at risk of contracting TB.

While public health experts of a century ago failed to appreciate more casual means of tuberculosis transmission such as breathing and coughing, they did, at least, understand that TB was communicable from one person to another. In order to prevent the spread of disease to others, most physicians and public health workers agreed it was essential to both report new TB diagnoses to the local or state health authorities and to isolate seriously afflicted individuals.

Yet the biases and prejudices of the day framed many of these public health policies. Several tuberculosis-reporting regulations of this era were distinctly shaped by the assumption that it was the lower classes who posed the greatest threat to the public health. Thus, privately practicing physicians who treated the well-to-do were generally not required to report their tuberculosis patients to the public authorities while doctors working at free clinics, dispensaries, and other institutions that catered to the poor were. Many poor or immigrant patients either avoided doctors entirely or sought out quacks who at least promised confidentiality. More productively, charities and immigrant aid societies opened and operated TB clinics staffed by their own physicians in an effort to comply with the public health laws of the land while assisting these people.[34]

Around this time a number of Americans grew steadily obsessed with the threat of allowing TB- and other germ-ridden immigrants into the United States. One was a wealthy, balding, and painfully thin Boston attorney named Prescott Farnsworth Hall who served as the secretary of the Immigration Restriction League from 1894 to 1921.[35] Beginning in the late 1890s, Hall and his supporters lobbied to make contagious diseases like trachoma and favus (a fungal skin rash) causes for exclusion. Well aware of how few immigrants would actually be excluded for such illnesses, he next turned to the matter of body type. Hall argued that the "poor physiques" of immigrants, such as East European Jewish tailors who had deformed posture as a result of hunching over sewing machines, would cause nothing but problems. Such "physical degenerates" were "not only unlikely to become a desirable citizen, but also very likely to transmit his undesirable qualities [to others]."[36] By 1907, several federal immigration acts included these conditions in the medical exclusion categories, but in actual numbers of those rejected these statutes did little to stem the torrential tide of immigrants coming to America during these years.

As a result, Prescott Hall attempted to link the "poor physique" strategy to the contagious threat of imported tuberculosis.[37] Although several prominent doctors observed that the incidence of tuberculosis among immigrants was significantly lower than that of native-born Americans, Hall actively publicized a tuberculosis-immigrant connection. During the first two decades of the twentieth century, Hall warned that allowing "poorly-built" immigrants would result in an epidemic of tuberculosis that would ruin the fragile American health care and charitable systems, not to mention the health of its people.[38]

One example of this physical restriction was the case of a nineteen-year-old man named Supermoney Munsammy from Madras, India, who was diagnosed at Ellis Island as "a dwarf with curvature of the spine." In fact, Munsammy came to America with a contract as a performer in the Ringling Brothers and Barnum & Bailey Circus. He appeared in that venue's "Freak Show" as a highly regarded and popular contortionist during the 1901–1903 seasons before returning to India. Munsammy subsequently decided to rejoin the circus for the 1910 season. Among those testifying on his behalf at his special board of inquiry hearing at Ellis Island on March 16, 1910, was John Ringling. The legendary showman assured the U.S. government that his production company would house, observe, and take full responsibility for Munsammy during the circus's performing season and return him to India at the end of the year. Despite this high-profile appeal, Munsammy was judged to be so physically deformed under the "poor physique" statute and "likely to become a public charge" as a potential tuberculosis victim that the immigration authorities ordered him deported immediately.[39]

Ultimately, episodic battles with epidemics were simply not enough to inspire permanent immigration restriction laws. Instead, Hall and the immigration restrictionists turned to the authoritative language of eugenics and inherited deleterious traits to make their case. Diseased newcomers, they effectively argued, not only threatened the public health in the present because of their propensity toward acute illness and poverty; they also threatened the future of American society as they passed on their defective genes in multiplicity, generation after generation. A major result of this strategy was the Immigration Restriction Act of 1924, one of the widest-reaching and ethnically biased immigration restriction statutes on the federal books. Not surprisingly, particular types of immigrants were legislated to be the most objectionable: East European Jews, southern Italians, Balkans, Turks, Greeks, Asians, and Arabs.[40] Ironically, Prescott Hall never lived to see the Immigration Restriction Act that he had worked so hard to develop pass into law. Long in "poor health" and, according to his wife, "a frail, little hothouse plant," Hall died in 1921 after a "long and tedious illness" at the age of fifty-three. These descriptions were euphemisms for the ultimate cause of his demise: tuberculosis.[41]

One hallmark of the treatment of tuberculosis during the first half of the twentieth century was an enforced and long-term stay in a sanatorium (from the Latin, "a house where one went to be cured"). Today, most people who think about tuberculosis sanatoria at all recall bucolic, woodsy facilities such as the famed Saranac Lake Sanatorium in the Adirondack Mountains, which catered to patients like Robert Louis Stevenson and the New York Giants pitching ace Christy Mathewson. To be sure, there were many facilities that provided excellent care at a premium price, the Betty Ford Clinics of their time. But these small private sanatoria that catered to the rich could never hope to serve the tens of thousands of tuberculosis-afflicted Americans, and there existed a wide range of isolation facilities across the United States matching the medical, economic, and social circumstances of their clients.[42]

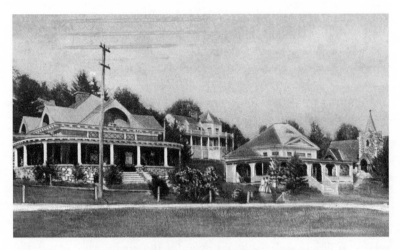

*The Saranac Tuberculosis Sanatorium in the*
*Adirondack Mountains, in upstate New York*

Regardless of the social standing of their clientele, the tuberculosis
sanatoria were firmly guided by all kinds of rules: how to act, sleep,
dress, exercise, what and when to eat, and even whom to associate with.
Relationships between men and women patients were strictly forbidden.[43] Patients had to endure weekly weigh-ins to make sure that the TB
was being held in check rather than "consuming" their bodies. Those
who failed to improve with the help of the prescribed dietary and fresh
air regimens were often transferred to an "incurables" facility so as not to
diminish the "cure rate" of a particular sanatorium, which was an essential attraction to recruiting new and paying customers.[44]

Whether one was cured at a tuberculosis sanatorium or not, there was
a definite public health benefit to these institutions. Decades before the
advent of antibiotics in 1947, physicians observed a striking decrease in
the incidence of tuberculosis in Europe and the United States. By 1923,
the eminent British public health official Sir Arthur Newsholme theorized that the decline of TB in his country resulted from reduced exposure to infection brought about by the segregation of impoverished and
immigrant consumptives in Poor Law infirmaries.[45] This same trend was
noted in the United States during this period. The more tuberculosis

sanatoria or isolation hospitals in operation, the greater the potential for those with the infection to be removed from the healthy. The result was a steady decline in cases that only accelerated with the advent of the powerful anti-tuberculosis drugs that began to be used in the late 1940s.[46]

There is, of course, a huge cost to such isolation for those who find themselves separated from their loved ones. Those fortunate enough to live among the healthy rarely give this thorny side of quarantine a second thought. It is simply a requirement for maintaining the public health. But those who are isolated understand the cost of imposed loneliness all too well. With tuberculosis, this experience was magnified by the fact that most sanatoria were situated far away from urban centers both to discourage all contact with visitors and the outside world and to promote a stress-free and complete rest, albeit within a decidedly gloomy atmosphere of illness and death. Yet even for those who were cured, the stigma of disease was hard to shake. Thirty years after her stay at a Colorado sanatorium during World War II, a nurse named Iva Marie Lowry recalled: "There are some of us without blemish or without breaking a law of society that are still as much of an outcast as he who robbed or murdered. One enters a jail; the other enters a sanatorium. Each comes out 'branded for life.' "[47]

The stigma of tuberculosis that continues to thrive decades after the last sanatorium closed its doors is well illustrated by the experiences of a fifty-two-year-old Ethiopian immigrant and patient named Abdul, whom I met at the New York–Presbyterian Hospital Tuberculosis Clinic. A short, compact man with thinning, jet black hair, Abdul is a natty dresser and charming conversationalist. He came to the interview in a carefully arranged outfit of a plaid sports jacket, white vest, and woolen pants that were precisely pressed, pleated, and cuffed. Abdul reminded me of my grandfather; they were among the few men I have known who always pinched the crease of their pant legs as they sat down to ensure they looked equally good in the seated and the standing positions. Abdul's dark complexion and accented English were eliciting stares of suspicion since the fateful September day the jetliners crashed into the three landmark buildings. With a spirit of good cheer that I was to learn framed his entire outlook of the world, Abdul added: "But I can handle it. Look, I've had to get used to people's reactions when I tell them I am being treated for tuberculosis. It could be much worse, you know." Abdul added, "My brother's name is Jihad."

Abdul came from a well-to-do prominent family of landowners. He was trained as a schoolteacher in Ethiopia with a specialty in accounting and business administration, and taught briefly before joining the Ethiopian Ministry of Education in the late 1960s. During the 1970s he became active in the protest movement against the rule of Emperor Haile Selassie. In the early spring of 1972, several friends who were also involved in these protests were harassed and one was beaten to death, inspiring Abdul to take a long trip to the United States on a tourist's visa.

He left Ethiopia in July 1972 on an El-Al flight that stopped first in Tel Aviv. Abdul explained that his choice of airline was based on "the terrific fares they were offering at the time." Coincidentally, that same month, terrorists from the Palestinian Liberation Organization murdered eleven Israeli athletes at the Olympic Games in Munich. Almost thirty years later, Abdul still recalled the intense scrutiny and suspicion he was subjected to during his stopover in Tel Aviv.

His first months in America were baffling, and it took him a while to adjust to the hectic pace of New York City. By the late fall of 1972, Abdul decided he wanted to live there permanently. He applied for and obtained a green card, and embarked on a series of jobs including clerical worker in a brokerage firm, office manager in a lawyer's office, and taxicab driver on the weekends. He also attended evening classes at the City University of New York from 1977 to 1986, and graduated with a Bachelor of Science degree in economics. But the proudest day of his life, Abdul beamed, was "when I was naturalized as an American citizen on July 4, 1990."

In late 1992, Abdul's mother became seriously ill, and because his father had long since died, he returned to Ethiopia to help his brother Jihad, a prosperous businessman, care for her. Abdul lived in Ethiopia for the next six years when he began to feel tired and complain of difficulty breathing. In the months that followed, Abdul consulted "the finest doctors at our most expensive, prestigious hospitals." After each medical consultation, he returned home without relief, let alone cure.

In May 1999, one of his physicians told Abdul that he probably had a "mild case" of tuberculosis but failed to order an X-ray or prescribe the anti-tuberculosis medications he required. Abdul was astonished by the diagnosis and for several days clung to the hope that the doctor was reading from the wrong chart: "I never thought *I* would contract tuberculosis. My brother was even more upset than I was. He screamed at the doctor 'How can this possibly be? Only poor people get TB.' "

Growing more and more ill with each passing week, Abdul decided to return to the United States for treatment. On July 11, he purchased a one-way ticket to Newark International Airport, and his plane landed on the tarmac a little after noon the following day. Because he was an American citizen with a valid passport, he had no trouble going through customs even though, as he later recalled, "I was so sick I could not believe that someone did not at least stop me to see what was going on. I could barely walk, let alone carry my bags, and I could not stop coughing.

"I couldn't eat. I had absolutely no appetite, and the pounds were, literally, melting off of my body," Abdul continued. "My color was awful. Each night I woke up in a pool of sweat, and I finally stopped wearing pajamas because it was as if someone poured a bucket of water on me while I was sleeping." Drenching night sweats, incidentally, are definitive harbingers of serious illness. So ominous is this symptom, I often instruct medical students that when your patient complains of night sweats, *you* should begin sweating too.

Within two days of his arrival, his niece put him in a taxicab with explicit instructions to the driver to take him to New York–Presbyterian Hospital. In the emergency room, an X-ray of his chest provided a definitive answer behind Abdul's copious night sweats, hacking cough, and paralyzing fatigue: he had a huge cavitary lesion in the top of his left lung, a finding that screamed pulmonary tuberculosis.

Soon after being informed of this diagnosis, Abdul was whisked to an isolation room, where gowned, gloved, and masked doctors and nurses poked and prodded to extract blood, urine, spinal fluid, and a biopsy of his liver. Fortunately, only his lungs were involved, and the strain of tuberculosis he was infected with was responsive to antibiotics. Nevertheless, he remained contagious to others for almost four weeks after initiating treatment, and was required to endure elaborate isolation procedures including wearing a special face mask to prevent the spread of TB germs to others. When we met, Abdul's doctor boasted about his complete recovery from the brink of death only a few years earlier. But once she left the room, Abdul admitted that despite the striking improvement in his physical health, the psychological stigma of tuberculosis is something he continues to struggle with:

> A lot of my friends did not want to visit me in the hospital. My niece—a girl I helped raise—told my doctor, *not me,* that I was not welcome to return to her

apartment when I was discharged. She has not spoken to me since she found out that her nine-year-old boy, my grandnephew, tested positive for TB. Even though he is okay now, I still feel terrible. For months, I stayed awake at night crying that I would no longer be accepted in society. More than the loneliness, the exhaustion, the disease itself, the real pain comes from the guilt I continue to feel about my nephew and God knows who else. I mean, how many other people have been infected with tuberculosis because of me?

D r. William Osler, one of the founding physicians of the famed Johns Hopkins Hospital and the author of the most influential textbook on medicine of the late nineteenth and early twentieth centuries, understood quite a bit about tuberculosis and even more about human behavior. In 1894, Dr. Osler reminded the throng of students and doctors paying rapt attention to his every word: "the desire to take medicine is perhaps the greatest feature which distinguishes man from animals."[48] Most physicians today would amend Osler's observation. To wit: human beings are willing and eager to "take medicine," provided that there are few side effects and the course of treatment is brief. Both additions to this famous medical axiom are particularly germane to the modern treatment of tuberculosis.

Throughout the 1930s a soil microbiologist named Selman Waksman studied a fungus named *Streptomyces griseus* that prefers to reside in compost heaps, peat bogs, and piles of manure. One day in 1939, while tinkering away in his laboratory at Rutgers University, Waksman observed that when the fungus was placed in the same culture dish with colonies of bacteria, the fungus inhibited or halted altogether the growth of the bacteria. We now understand that the ability for microorganisms to have the means to kill one another is a perversely critical act of life. Without such naturally occurring antibiotics, the planet's surface would soon be buried by a mountain range of germs!

It was Waksman and his colleagues who first isolated the chemical compounds in *Streptomyces griseus* that could be used to combat infection. Many of these substances had a wide range of toxic side effects unacceptable for use in humans. But one compound, streptomycin, discovered in 1943, seemed to fit the bill. Working with a team of doctors at the Mayo Clinic, Waksman went through a herd of guinea pigs before finally using it on human beings with tuberculosis. The drug proved so effective that in 1944 the research team gleefully announced they had discovered a "magic bullet" that would finally free human civilization from the destructive power of consumption.[49]

Ultimately, streptomycin did not turn out to be as definitive a cure for TB as initially predicted. Soon after its isolation, however, microbiologists discovered a number of other anti-tuberculosis medications that proved to be far more effective. Most Americans promptly concluded that these drugs were the final nails in TB's coffin. The statistics of decline were, in fact, convincing. In 1944, before anti-tuberculosis drugs were introduced, there were 130,000 new cases of tuberculosis in the United States; in 1989 there were fewer than 24,000 cases.[50] Yet while most doctors were making firm declarations of victory over the white plague, there were some warnings to the contrary. Shortly after winning the Nobel Prize for his work in 1952, Dr. Waksman presciently worried that the "problems of resistance resulting in the recurrence of the disease might obliterate any potentialities that streptomycin might have for the treatment of the disease."[51] Other tuberculosis experts cautioned about these risks as well. Sadly, few of us paid attention to the threat of drug-resistant infections until very recently.

Now, if the treatment of tuberculosis were confined to simply taking a few pills for a few days, releasing its grip on humanity might be a relatively simple matter. Alas, mycobacteria are not all that easy to kill. To begin with, antibiotics have a difficult time penetrating their hard, waxy cell wall coats. Another problem arises from the fact that germs are most vulnerable to antibiotic annihilation when they are multiplying. A germ such as *Streptococcus*, a common cause of pneumonia, reproduces itself every twenty minutes or so, but TB germs at their most fecund multiply only every twenty-four hours. Moreover, mycobacteria have the ability to go into a somewhat dormant state for long periods of time and the anti-tuberculosis drugs we prescribe actually decrease these germs' already slow growth rate. As a result of all these biological characteristics, a patient with tuberculosis must take antibiotics for months. At present, the standard treatment is a six-month regimen consisting of daily doses of three different anti-tuberculosis drugs. This task may sound easy to the doctor writing the prescription, but it is one that almost always loses something in the translation.

Today we would refer to what Dr. Osler described as the innately human "desire to take medicine" as "patient compliance." But here's the rub: most humans are not terribly compliant with regard to taking extended courses of medicine, especially once they no longer feel ill. Even patients with severe tuberculosis start to feel remarkably better after a few weeks of treatment. As a result of this incredible turnaround, many simply stop taking their medication even though such a decision almost always means a relapse of disease and frequently sets the scene for their developing drug resistance.[52]

Compliance becomes even more difficult when a patient suffers from alcoholism, depression, drug addiction, or is homeless. And, of course, the failure to follow a doctor's orders to the letter plagues every sector of human society. There is a prodigious body of medical literature attesting to the fact that regardless of educational attainment, wealth, race, ethnicity, or gender, the little prescription vials we joyfully take home from the pharmacy are rarely emptied to completion. Many people—including doctors—don't finish a ten-day course of antibiotics for strep throat, let alone the six-month regimen necessary for tuberculosis.[53] There also exist several unpleasant side effects with anti-TB medications that can contribute to noncompliance, such as their propensity to turn one's urine the color of orange soda pop or to cause intense nausea, abdominal pain, visual problems, allergic reactions, rashes, and hepatitis.

Regardless of the reason, when these medications are taken irregularly or discontinued after a few weeks or months, the risk for encouraging drug-resistant strains only increases. In these cases, the germs that tend to survive best are those that carry drug-resistant traits. Hence, incomplete treatment can actually nurture the resistant strains while killing off the sensitive ones. The result is a new, drug-resistant case of tuberculosis that is extremely difficult to treat, necessitates several far more expensive and toxic medications, and can require twenty-four months or longer for treatment. In many cases multidrug-resistant tuberculosis is incurable, making this essentially "man-made phenomenon" one of the most serious threats to the world's health today.[54]

To avert this problem, most public health workers now advocate "directly observed therapy" programs (DOTS) where a member of a health care team observes patients taking their daily doses of medication. The actual ingestion of pills can take place in a clinic, in the patient's home, or a mutually agreed upon location. These programs have been extraordinarily successful in treating and controlling the spread of tuberculosis and promoting these patients' general health. But they do not come cheap. The average cost of care per patient is about $6,000. This figure seems entirely reasonable, however, when compared to the cost of caring for someone who develops the multidrug-resistant version of tuberculosis. Their medical bills skyrocket to at least $200,000 per patient in 2002 dollars.

One might look to the recent history of tuberculosis in New York City over the past forty years to appreciate the value of such an investment. In the late 1960s the New York City Department of Health spent over $41 million each year on tuberculosis treatment and prevention programs, including twenty-four specialized TB clinics based around the city, tuberculosis wards in the public hospitals, and hundreds of specially trained TB caseworkers. As a result of these efforts, new TB cases declined steadily in the city each year between 1960 and 1978.[55]

Basking in the glow of overconfidence and changing budget priorities, New York City began to execute massive funding cuts for almost every public health program, especially those directed at tuberculosis control. For example, in 1978 the city spent only $2 million on tuberculosis control. By 1980, the city employed 10 outreach workers to respond to the 8,000-plus new or suspected cases of tuberculosis a year. Instead of 1,000 tuberculosis-designated hospital beds, there were now only 100. Added to this volatile mix were two decades of increasing numbers of homeless Americans, the dismantling of psychiatric and public hospitals, the rise of HIV/AIDS, and the boom in immigration from nations where TB is common. Each of these factors helped to create a situation one infectious disease expert has labeled a "tuberculosis time bomb."[56]

In 1979 the decades-long decline in tuberculosis in New York City came to an abrupt end, and by 1992, the TB case rate ballooned to almost three times what it was in 1979. More striking, doctors established that once released from the hospital, only 11 percent of tuberculosis patients completed their six-month course of medication and that one out of every three newly diagnosed cases in the city was multidrug resistant.[57]

In response, the health department unrolled a massive anti-tuberculosis campaign, including neighborhood TB screening programs, DOTS clinics, improved health care in the city's jails, and for noncompliant patients a special detention (or quarantine) facility whose very existence seemed to encourage patients to "comply with less restrictive treatments." The price tag for these interventions was more than $1 billion. For the present, the tide appears to have turned in New York. In the years following the epidemic's peak in 1992, multidrug-resistant cases of TB in New York City fell by 91 percent, and the overall TB case rate fell from a high of 49.8 cases per 100,000 to 16.6 cases per 100,000. Nevertheless, this incidence remains almost three times the nationwide rate of 5.8 cases per 100,000.[58]

Today, few public health experts are quick to claim victory over tuberculosis, and many remain deeply worried that the white plague will rear its ugly head once again with disastrous results. The problem is getting the rest of the population to listen. Indeed, it is the complacence factor, the too quick impulse we have to forget about the public health threats that incited intense panic only weeks or a month before that has these professionals most concerned. Hopefully we have learned that the most costly disruptions to a community's health invariably take place when the programs we so easily take for granted are halted—even for brief periods.[59]

In 2002 tuberculosis in the United States was declared to be at an all-time low. From its peak incidence of 26,673 newly diagnosed cases in 1992, it has fallen to 16,377 cases. Similarly, the rate of multidrug-resistant cases of TB has fallen by 70 percent. Still of concern is that 50 percent of the TB cases diagnosed each year are among the foreign-born, compared to 27 percent in 1992. But these numbers require scrutiny before we blithely blame immigrants for the problem. In fact, the actual number of foreign-born people diagnosed in the United States each year has been fairly constant over the past decade (about 8,000 cases a year between 1992 and 2000) while the number of American-born cases has decreased markedly. This suggests that most tuberculosis cases among the foreign-born in the United States are due to the reactivation of latent disease—infections these people may have contracted months or years ago but without suffering any real symptoms or actual disease—as opposed to the transmission of new cases. The solution, then, is to develop programs that identify and treat those with latent tuberculosis infections around the world.[60]

Despite the success in our own country, there should be no illusions: the crisis remains real. TB is still with us and stronger than ever, especially in the former USSR, China, the Caribbean, Africa, and South and Central America, where both forms of tuberculosis, drug sensitive and multidrug resistant, are rampant. Ninety-five percent of all cases of tuberculosis occur among impoverished residents in developing countries. These circumstances require creative innovations in treatment and prevention programs, especially for multidrug-resistant TB; new developments in our scientific understanding of the disease; significant economic and human resources that are carefully applied and consistently replenished; and international cooperation as cultures and nations meld their work into a global effort. By working to detect at least 70 percent of all tuberculosis cases and cure 85 percent of all patients identified around the world, we could save about 16 million lives by 2010.[61] But in order to accomplish this, we must accept that we will never completely conquer tuberculosis—or probably any other infectious disease for that matter. The best we can hope for is to contain it enough to limit its influence.

# TWO

# Bubonic Plague Visits
# San Francisco's Chinatown

[On the morning the Health Department announced the quarantine] the white employers of the Chinese awoke to find that there was nobody on hand to prepare breakfast. The chef at the Palace Hotel waited in vain for the dozen or more Chinese under his orders to appear, and a similar state of affairs developed in nearly every place where Chinese were employed. The central telephone in Chinatown was kept busy for hours making connections for angry citizens who were trying to get a trace of missing servants. Chinese stores were open, only to be closed again when proprietors learned that trouble of an unknown character had befallen the place. Chinese by the score braved the anger of police officers and tried to make their way outside and though some of them were shoved back abruptly, others would journey to the ropes, only to receive like treatment.

—"Nothing but a Suspicion," *San Francisco Chronicle,* March 8, 1900[1]

In 1900 thousands of bedraggled newcomers were arriving at Ellis Island every day, and droves of them settled in squalid, overcrowded tenements in cities like New York, Boston, Philadelphia, and Baltimore. Yet despite the predictions of many Americans, the first immigrant-associated epidemic of the twentieth century did not occur along the Atlantic seaboard or in its teeming ghettos. Instead, a mysterious outbreak of bubonic plague unfolded more than three thousand miles away in San Francisco. During the course of human history, few epidemic diseases have elicited more fear than bubonic plague, and the San Francisco episode proved to be no exception. But added to the unsavory mix of contagion, death, and panic were human vectors who belonged to a group many Americans considered to be the most foreign and dangerous of the new arrivals: Chinese immigrants.

Bubonic plague is caused by a tiny, rod-shaped bacterium named *Yersinia pestis*. Before the development of antibiotics and depending on the virulence of the germ itself, anywhere from 35 to 90 percent of those who encountered the germ died a miserable death. More than two thousand years ago it probably descended from a benign, gut-dwelling bacterium named *Yersinia pseudotuberculosis*. An infection of the less lethal version of *Yersinia* merely generates an annoying stomachache. But in an evolutionary blink of the eye, a period of only a few hundred years or so, *Yersinia pestis* somehow learned to leap between fleas and mammals and to thrive in the blood rather than the intestine. The result

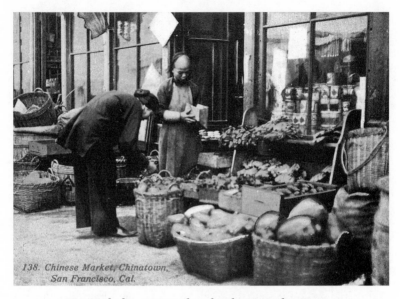

138. Chinese Market, Chinatown, San Francisco, Cal.

*During the late nineteenth and early twentieth centuries, Chinese immigrants were one of the groups Americans considered to be the most foreign and dangerous.*

was the aggressive and easily spread illness we now recognize as "the plague," the cause of millions of deaths over the past two millennia.

Across this time span there have been three major pandemics: *Antiqua*, which occurred during the reign of Emperor Justinian and lasted from 500 to 700; *Medievalis*, which gave rise to the notorious pandemic during the fourteenth century, swept through Asia, North Africa, the Middle East, and Europe, and rampaged well into the seventeenth century; and *Orientalis*, which began in the late nineteenth century in the south of China and continues to be the cause of some four thousand deaths a year. Today, there is much deliberation among medical historians about whether each of these pandemics was caused solely by *Yersinia* or a combination of deadly pathogens, such as smallpox, typhus, influenza, anthrax, acute diarrheal diseases, *and* plague. Such musings serve as excellent proof of one of the great benefits of finding work as an epidemiologist of the past: there is always room for debate and, given the lack of definitive evidence, new theories.

Regardless of their exact cause, these visitations were known by many ominous and uninviting names, such as the Black Death, the Great Mortality, and the Universal Plague. They decimated entire cities and regions, leaving stacks of bodies in their wakes. Between 1347 and 1351 alone, 33 percent or more of Europe's population died from the *Medievalis* strain of the plague. Those fortunate enough to avoid the initial waves of infection often fled to other parts of the nations they inhabited, but unwittingly brought the deadly germ with them.

Some of the earliest known quarantine laws were developed during the fourteenth century in response to the Black Death. The very word "quarantine" was derived from the Italian *quarante giorni,* or forty days, and *quarantenaria* was the name of the public health edict handed down in Venice in 1374. At the first sign of bubonic plague's approach, the gates or port of a city were literally shut tight for a period of forty days, which was believed by Renaissance physicians to be the amount of time required for plague to burn itself out. Perhaps more chilling, bubonic plague may well have been used as one of the first biological weapons. In 1347, while attacking the Genoese-controlled Black Sea port of Caffa, the Tartars hurled bodies of their plague victims over the city walls in order to spread the disease among their enemies.

Bubonic plague is a flea-borne disease; most mammals that contract the Black Death are bitten by these pesky insects that have already encountered the germ. However, not all fleas are equal. Because the anatomy of the gastrointestinal tract of a few species of fleas is more amenable to the multiplication of *Yersinia* than other varieties, some fleas are, in essence, better plague spreaders than others. For example, *Pulex cheopis,* the Oriental or Indian rat flea that predominates in Asia, Africa, and South America, is far more voracious and efficient at delivering deadly germs than the northern European rat flea, *Ceratophyllus fasciatus.*

The major mammal reservoir for *Yersinia* around the globe is the wild rodent population. Although more than three hundred different species have been implicated, the favored victim appears to be the animal biologists call *Rattus rattus* and most everyone else simply refers to as the black rat. Unlike rabbits, prairie dogs, or squirrels, which not only survive encounters with *Yersinia* but also continue to reproduce while infected, rats that contract the plague typically die in a matter of days to weeks. Occasionally, rats—both infected and healthy—travel farther than intended, especially if they live near a seaport. To this day, oceangoing vessels have metal cones or discs on their mooring ropes called rat catchers, which were created as a means of preventing most intrepid rodents from climbing aboard, stowing away, and spreading disease.

Wherever they are found, plague-infected rats can be a public health nightmare. Anyone assigned the unseemly (and downright dangerous) task of examining a plague-ridden rat carcass will all too readily recount their memorably disgusting findings, especially the dead rodent's wide-open, glazed-over eyes and the oozing, bloody ulcers that mar its coat. As these dead rats repose in an alleyway or field, droves of hungry fleas descend upon their bodies in search of a meal of coagulated blood. But when there are not enough rats, or other rodents, to feast upon, the infection-carrying fleas fly off to find other warm-blooded bodies—any mammalian species will do—in search of another snack. As a result of our evolving understanding of the *Yersinia* germ's travel habits, public health experts no longer advocate exterminating all rats in a particular community at once. To illustrate, if the Pied Piper of Hamlin were to ply his trade at the wrong point during a bubonic plague epidemic, the total disappearance of a rodent reservoir might actually increase the likelihood of human involvement because the bloodthirsty fleas would have no rats to prey upon.

Indeed, it is precisely at this moment in the complex life cycle of *Yersinia pestis* that human beings enter the story. Instead of rats or other burrowing rodents, the infected fleas bite a human and leave behind their plague-riddled feces and saliva. The unsuspecting human typically notices only an itchy sensation and then scratches his skin, making a tiny but entirely adequate entry point for the microbe. Before anyone knows it, *Yersinia* has a new host. When *Yersinia pestis* does commingle with a human population, it often spreads quickly, and the death rates can be staggering. This is especially so where no attempts are made to isolate the ill and selectively exterminate rats and fleas, and access to reliable medical interventions such as antibiotics is poor.

The incubation period of plague, the time between initial infection and descent into a pathological hell, can be anywhere between two and fifteen days, with the average time being six days. Raging fevers, accompanied by intense aches in the muscles and head, an unendurable sense of exhaustion, and bloody vomiting characterize the first rings of the plague's inferno. This agony is soon followed by the appearance of painful, rock-hard, swollen lymph glands called buboes, derived from the Greek word for "groin." But the groin is hardly *Yersinia*'s only destination. Any lymph gland—in the neck, armpit, elbow, or elsewhere in the body—is an enticing site for the microbe to set up shop.

Lymph glands, or nodes, which are connected by lithe byways or channels that traverse the body almost in parallel to the more robust circulatory system, help filter and trap invading organisms that have somehow gained entry. They also contribute to the production of white blood cells called lymphocytes, some of the most potent soldiers in the body's guard patrol against the relentless invasion by microbes. In the case of an infection with plague, however, the *Yersinia* germs multiply at such an astounding rate that they clog the victim's lymph nodes, rendering them useless. Such a haven for propagation is a brilliantly perverse microbiologic coup d'état. Not only do these fecund and deadly germs compromise the entity responsible for making cells that might kill them, but their favored anatomical way stations also provide easy access, via the lymph channels and bloodstream, to other parts in the body. Hence, a crop of buboes is one of the best indicators that plague germs have reproduced frenetically and traveled extensively through the body.

Almost everyone who has experienced a sore throat and its attendant swollen lymph nodes can attest to the pain this sensation engenders. Yet buboes, *Yersinia pestis*–filled nodes, are *not* merely swollen glands. Often the size of a small piece of fruit or even a baseball, these fluid-filled pockets of germs, pus, and inflammation cause a pain that is unbearable. Indeed, it is so intense that many victims of past eras begged their physicians to cut the buboes open, hoping these swellings would drain and the excruciating pressure would be relieved. Sadly, such a maneuver offers only temporary relief. No knife, no matter how skillfully wielded by a surgeon, is a match for the *Yersinia*. In fact, lancing a bubo open only allows still another highway for the germ's spread because it affords a superb opportunity for *Yersinia* to exit a swollen node and to enter the autobahn of the bloodstream. In their wake, these microbes leave behind a telltale trail of blood clots and bruises, called petechiae, that bubble from deep within the capillaries, venules, and arterioles and up into the skin's surface as they damage more and more of the victim's inner organs.

For those attending to the needs of a plague-stricken victim, the most frightening aspect of the job is looking at the patient's face. The nostrils angrily flare outward. The eyes become sunken, the pupils dilate with a vengeance—an appearance doctors often refer to as "doll's eyes"—and the patient's face typically wears an intensely anxious expression. It is a look that many have described as the realization by the victim that he or she is about to experience a horrific death.

If this scenario isn't terrifying enough, there exists an even more virulent variant of the disease called pneumonic plague, where *Yersinia* microbes travel directly through the air into the victim's lungs. As the lungs rapidly fill with the germ's deadly progeny, merely coughing and exhaling in the presence of others can now transmit the plague. The healthy person then inhales the microbes and soon after dies a miserable death. One recent case in 1992 illustrated this phenomenon all too well: in Colorado, a veterinarian died within hours after an infected cat sneezed on him while he was trying to rescue the feline from underneath a house. Bypassing the slower (and in a public health sense, more easily controlled) vector of rats and fleas, pneumonic plague is among the most unmanageable epidemic diseases known.[2]

The opening scene of the San Francisco bubonic plague epidemic began just after midnight on March 6, 1900, in the basement of a dilapidated boardinghouse pretentiously named the Globe Hotel. Around this time one of the Globe's guests wondered why the moaning man sleeping next to him was suddenly mute. This concerned boarder, whose name is lost, had been glad enough he had the requisite ten cents to sleep inside on that cold and damp night. But unlike his fellow roommates, about forty or fifty Chinese immigrants much like himself, he became more and more troubled by the silence of a fellow countryman he had never met and would never know.

Rousing himself out of bed and reflexively dusting the dirt and bedbugs off his wrinkled clothing, he padded over to the once-whimpering man's cot. He did not have far to travel. Flophouses like the Globe, present in almost every slum neighborhood of every American city, were a common source of housing for newly arrived immigrants and the urban poor. They were notorious for their overcrowding, foul smells, and decidedly unhealthy conditions.[3]

Even to one uninitiated in the art of medical diagnosis, the silent man was clearly dead. Foamy, blood-tinged spittle covered his lips, his skin was ashen gray and cold to the touch, and, under the threadbare blanket that covered his naked body, there were baseball-sized swellings around his groin and armpits. The Chinese lodger who made this unsettling discovery alerted the hotel's night clerk. After looking up the cot number in his register book, the clerk announced that the deceased man was a forty-one-year-old named Chick Gin and immediately telephoned the city health department. Although the Chinese community of San Francisco preferred their own doctors and undertakers to the American variety, local law mandated that the city pathologist examine anyone who died unattended by a physician or under mysterious circumstances.[4]

Soon after Chick Gin's body was delivered to the city morgue early that morning, it was placed on a marble table in the autopsy suite. There, it awaited an examination many physicians fondly refer to as "the doctor's final court of appeals." The pathologist, a young man only one year out of medical school named Frank P. Wilson, began with a procedure that has been used to examine the dead for centuries: a careful inspection for lesions of the skin, swellings, and other external evidence that might explain the patient's death. Wilson followed this search by picking up a razor-sharp scalpel and making a deep Y-shaped cut into the corpse's torso, with the short arms of the Y extending from the ends of the collarbone and its central trunk going down the middle of the chest and abdomen, ending at the groin. Such invasion affords a wide enough entry into the body to be able to examine what the surgeon and writer Sherwin Nuland has eloquently termed "the mysteries within."[5]

As Dr. Wilson explored the swollen and blood-engorged inner organs in the deep recesses of Chick Gin's pelvis, he became convinced that this was no ordinary death. The young pathologist urgently asked his assistant to call the senior health officer, Dr. A. P. O'Brien, and the city bacteriologist, Wilfred Kellogg, out of their beds at home and into the autopsy suite as soon as possible. And while we have no record of their arrival an hour or so later, they were likely flabbergasted. The inflamed, distended lymph nodes throughout Chick Gin's dissected body and the microscopic slides smeared with these nodular remnants suggested an infectious disease that makes even the most brave and experienced physician shudder.

Given that bubonic plague was (and is) so rare in the United States, how did it come to San Francisco in 1900? Without specific culture or tissue samples, historians are forced to conjecture, but one theory seems particularly likely. In 1900, San Francisco was the ninth largest city in the United States, with a population of more than 300,000 and thousands more newcomers, both immigrants and native-born Americans from other parts of the nation, arriving each year. A sprawling, carelessly laid out city, San Francisco's fiscal health relied extensively on the commerce generated from the valued goods that arrived daily from the Far East through its port and "million dollar Ferry Building."[6]

Less welcome came a trickle of Chinese and even fewer Japanese, Korean, East Indian, and other Asian newcomers all lumped together by immigration officials under the heading "Orientals." The overwhelming majority of these immigrants were men who were farmers and unskilled laborers and either unmarried or leaving behind their wives in the hamlets of the Hsin-ning district of South China, near Canton. Like those forced to leave their homelands before and since, economic hardship and population pressures led to their migration from China to "Gold Mountain," the Chinese denomination for the United States.[7]

Beginning with the Chinese Exclusion Act of 1882 and a succession of statutes that curtailed their entry until the 1940s, the Chinese were the first immigrant group to be specifically excluded from entering the United States based on race. Those admitted under these laws were few in number, most typically students, teachers, government or diplomatic officials, travelers, the wives of merchants already living in the United States, and, under very specific circumstances, unskilled laborers. The statistical efficacy of these laws is clear: from 1848 to 1882 more than 250,000 Asian immigrants came to America; between 1882 and 1924 approximately 100,000 gained admission.[8] By comparison, 25 million immigrants from Eastern and Southern Europe came to the United States during this same period. A simple calculation reveals that Asians made up perhaps one-quarter of a percent of the total number of immigrants during the first great wave. The majority of them, approximately 75 percent, came through the port of San Francisco.[9]

Those most opposed to open immigration policies warned that allowing the Chinese to enter in the same proportion as European immigrants would lead only to disastrous results. Their warnings were widely accepted, and the majority of Americans justified these restrictions in a fervent belief that the Chinese were far more "foreign" and unassimilable than even the "new immigrants" from Europe. To be sure, the typical native-born American of 1900 feared the steady stream of Europe's "flotsam and jetsam" onto American shores. But many more viewed Chinese, Japanese, Korean, and Indian immigrants as completely foreign and dangerous to American society, evincing a racial separateness between white Americans and Asians that could never be blurred no matter how many coats of Americanization were painted on them.[10]

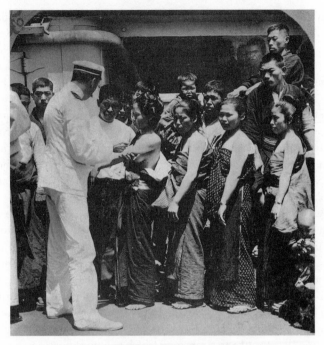

*Asian immigrants aboard a Pacific steamship bound
for Hawaii being vaccinated for smallpox, 1904*

During much of the nineteenth century isolated outbreaks of plague
occurred regularly in China, especially along the travel routes between
Canton, Hong Kong, and India. Disease control became especially difficult in 1892 when on the Manchurian frontier, muleteers and the animals that transported goods between Lianzhan and Yunnan were
discovered to be ill with plague. Always a hearty traveler, once the
microbe gained entry into this trade route, infected rats or people most
likely found passage on the junks that sailed between Canton and Hong
Kong, where the plague reached epidemic proportions in the mid-1890s,
and thence to British India. By 1895, it had struck Egypt, Japan, South
Africa, France, Great Britain, and Australia. In 1899 plague traveled as
far west as Oporto, Portugal, before crossing the Atlantic to Brazil.
Around the same time it migrated from China and Japan to Hawaii.[11]

On December 12, 1899, health officials in Honolulu announced that a twenty-two-year-old Chinese bookkeeper named You Chong had died of bubonic plague. Within hours after the discovery of his death, U.S. military police cordoned off the fourteen-square-block area where more than 10,000 Chinese and Japanese immigrants lived. A few weeks later, on January 20, 1900, Henry Cooper, the president of the Honolulu Board of Health, ordered a controlled burning of some of the buildings in this district to rid it of plague. As bad luck had it, a gust of wind quickly changed the fire's status to "uncontrolled," and the blaze spread throughout Honolulu's Chinatown, lasting a full seventeen days, laying ruin to over 4,000 homes across some 38 acres, and leaving 4,500 people homeless. Nevertheless, bubonic plague continued to appear episodically in Honolulu through early March 1900.[12]

It was probably around this time that *Yersinia* hitched a ride from China or Japan to San Francisco harbor in the bodies of rats stowing away in the many steamships that arrived weekly. What remains intriguing, however, is that Chick Gin was hardly a new arrival to San Francisco in 1900. He immigrated to the United States from Canton in 1884. During his last sixteen years he had lived in boardinghouses and earned a paltry living maintaining a woodshed where he sold scraps of lumber for fuel and household repairs. But somewhere in his travels through the slums and detritus of San Francisco, Chick Gin must have come in contact with either a plague-infected rat or flea.

W hen Drs. Wilson, O'Brien, and Kellogg first entertained their diagnosis of bubonic plague, they had only partial evidence to fully support such an assumption. While the gross appearance of Chick Gin's body, particularly his lymph glands, made for a strong case, more investigation was required before definitively linking the cause of death to *Yersinia*.

To make matters more complicated, Chick Gin's last weeks of life were not entirely consistent with the classic presentation of plague. Upon reading the next day's newspapers about the events at the Globe Hotel, a Chinese physician named Chung Bu Bing stepped forward to inform the health officials that he had been treating Chick Gin for a variety of complaints since January. None of Chick Gin's medical problems, his personal physician insisted, remotely resembled those of bubonic plague.

In fact, Chick Gin's physical complaints centered on severe pains in the head and the lower back, especially when urinating. Based on these symptoms, Dr. Chung Bu Bing thought the immigrant might be suffering from a bladder or urinary tract infection. On February 7 the doctor prescribed a Chinese herbal remedy with explicit instructions that Chick Gin return within seven days. However, the next week, on February 16, Chick Gin complained to a different physician, named Wong Ho, about painful and swollen lymph nodes and open sores near his groin and a foul-smelling discharge from the urethra, or opening, of his penis. In retrospect, this constellation of problems bears some resemblance to those seen in the sexually transmitted infection gonorrhea.[13]

While difficult to prove or disprove after all these years, a concurrent diagnosis of gonorrhea was entirely possible. Chick Gin, a single man who lived far away from his homeland, likely partook of the burgeoning prostitution trade in Chinatown. Most of the Chinese men living in San Francisco were prevented from marrying under the harshly restrictive Chinese immigration laws. Chinese women were often smuggled into the United States across the Mexican and Canadian borders or misrepresented as the wives of Chinese men already living in the United States only to become sex workers in one of the many brothels that operated in Chinatown. In 1900 there were approximately 2,200 Chinese women living in San Francisco, and at least 16 percent of them were prostitutes.[14]

At the end of February, Chick Gin was stricken by waves of severe vomiting and diarrhea, but he refused to seek additional medical attention. On the twenty-seventh he was described by one acquaintance as noticeably ill and in desperate need of some rest. Somehow, Chick Gin managed to obtain a cot in the basement of the Globe Hotel during the first days of March. By the sixth, however, he was dead. Among the many issues that needed to be sorted out by the doctors was whether Chick Gin's death was due to gonococcal sepsis (an overwhelming and deadly infection but, barring sexual contact, not terribly contagious to others), plague, or a combination of both.

If the diagnosis was, indeed, plague and the board of health had any hope of containing a potentially devastating epidemic, they would have to act fast. Dr. A. P. O'Brien announced to the press late in the afternoon of the sixth that the entire Chinese quarter should be cordoned off and quarantined while a bacteriologist conducted more extensive laboratory tests to prove or disprove the provisional diagnosis of bubonic plague. Many San Franciscans ridiculed this suggestion almost as soon as it was uttered. One reporter for the *San Francisco Chronicle* complained about the "harsh plan" whereby an entire city would be made to wait while a lone bacteriologist tinkered away with a dead man's body parts and experimental animals.[15]

The grousing of a steadily growing phalanx of journalists, politicians, and concerned observers belied the hard fact that physicians of any era rarely have precise understandings or solutions during the early stages of an epidemic. In 1900 doctors still relied heavily on their observations of a particular patient and broad clinical experience. What did the patient look like? What was his exact symptom pattern? What was the extent of his fever and at what point during the day did it reach its peak? Were any rashes or other clinical signs associated with fever? Did the disease appear to spread to others and how did it do so? All of these questions, and in most instances a good deal more, needed to be asked and answered to diagnose an infectious disease with any degree of confidence.

However, the San Francisco doctors were aided by the new and exciting bacteriological discoveries being made by scientists around the world. In 1894 two bacteriological investigators named Alexandre Yersin and Shibasaburo Kitasato, working independently in Hong Kong during the plague epidemic that year, identified a germ initially named *Bacillus pestis* and, later, *Yersinia pestis* as the cause of plague. So by 1900, while the science of epidemiology and bacteriology was far from perfect, physicians at least knew with some certainty that the *Yersinia* microbe was the etiologic cause of plague and what the germ looked like under the microscope. They were less certain, on the other hand, how plague spread from person to person and the roles played by rats and fleas.

In fact, the "harsh plan" of culturing germs from Chick Gin and then injecting them into laboratory animals for confirmation was not really harsh at all. It represented the cutting-edge scientific means of establishing a diagnosis of plague. The San Francisco physicians were simply following a set of scientific principles formulated by the world's premier bacteriologist, Dr. Robert Koch. Specifically, Koch's postulates instructed that in order to ascribe an infection to a particular bacterial organism, one first had to identify that organism in the diseased animal or person; second, isolate the organism in a pure culture; third, inoculate the cultured organism into a healthy animal; and finally, recover the putative organism from the experimental animal after it developed the disease in question. This rigorous process was essential given that a host of contaminating and non-disease-producing organisms could otherwise confuse a potential diagnosis and ruin the chances for an effective public health effort.[16]

Nor were the San Francisco doctors working alone. Dr. Walter Wyman, the surgeon general of the U.S. Marine Hospital Service (the forerunner to today's U.S. Public Health Service), dispatched assistant surgeon Joseph Kinyoun to help the San Francisco Health Department in their efforts to scientifically decipher Chick Gin's cause of death. In his time, Kinyoun was a major figure in the world of bacteriology. Often described as "industrious" and "hard working" rather than brilliant, he was, nevertheless, one of the best-trained bacteriologists in the United States.

In the 1880s, after medical studies at the St. Louis Medical College, Bellevue Hospital Medical College, and the Johns Hopkins University, the newly minted doctor Kinyoun traveled to Europe, where he studied bacteriology and laboratory technique under Robert Koch and several other eminent medical scientists. Upon his return in 1886, he joined the U.S. Marine Hospital Service and the following year founded the first bacteriological laboratory in the United States at the Marine Hospital on Staten Island, New York. With little more than a Zeiss microscope imported from Germany, a few culture plates, a Bunsen burner, and a tiny room in the basement of the hospital, Kinyoun established what ultimately grew into the National Institutes of Health. He helped introduce bacteriological methods for diagnosing cholera at the New York Quarantine Station in 1888 and, more famously, after his laboratory moved to Washington, D.C., in 1891, conducted an examination of the ventilation system of the U.S. House of Representatives. This latter study, published in 1894, concluded that the chamber was dangerously contaminated with illumination gas from leaking gas pipes and foul smells of tobacco expectoration saturating the carpets of the legislative chamber.[17]

In 1899 Kinyoun was reassigned as chief quarantine officer of San Francisco, either as the result of a fall from grace in the eyes of the surgeon general or in response to the looming threat of bubonic plague in China, Japan, and Hawaii. There he set up a bacteriology laboratory on Angel Island, the city's quarantine station located in San Francisco Bay, one mile south of the Tiburon Peninsula and forty minutes by boat from Fisherman's Wharf. Eleven years later, Angel Island became the "Ellis Island of the West" when the U.S. government officially designated it as an immigration reception station. As circumstances had it, Kinyoun did

not have to wait long for the Black Death to come knocking at his laboratory's door in the form of Chick Gin's disembodied lymph glands.

Although Dr. Kinyoun began to investigate Chick Gin's lymph glands
on March 7, he would not be able to arrive at any definite conclusion for
several days. But after the passage of a mere twenty-four hours, it was
clear that the natives of San Francisco were growing restless and wanted
an answer immediately. As one reporter for the *San Francisco Chronicle*
griped about the unavoidable delay, "A chattering monkey in the death
cell of the federal laboratory on Angel Island holds the fate of San Francisco within its mangy little hide."[18]

A maelstrom of controversy engulfed Kinyoun's work in the days
before the culture results could be interpreted. His most vituperative
critics accused him of being so medically incompetent that he was
unable to differentiate a simple case of pneumonia from bubonic plague
while those who supported his efforts counseled San Franciscans to be
calm and patient.[19] No matter what course of action Dr. Kinyoun chose,
however, he was bound to anger many members of the community. His
character flaws (he was often described as stubborn, argumentative, and
arrogant) and xenophobic beliefs (Kinyoun was known to have referred
to the Chinese as "Chinks" and to San Francisco as "Jew Town") only
escalated the remarkably difficult situation into a crisis of confidence in
the days and weeks that followed.

To most native-born Americans, Chinatown was at once foreign,
frightening, repugnant, fascinating, and exotic. Many wealthy San
Franciscans made trips to the Chinese neighborhood for entertainment
and in search of cheap labor. Others avoided the area entirely for fear of
contracting a disease or coming to some type of harm at the hands of the
"Yellow Menace." Chinatown was also home to a nefarious nightlife of
opium dens, gambling parlors, and bordellos that either attracted or
repelled San Franciscans, depending on their proclivities and moral
codes. The Chinese residents, on the other hand, had no real options to
live elsewhere and like many other newly arrived immigrant groups in
urban America of the early twentieth century, preferred living among
themselves out of fear of harassment, beatings, and other forms of abuse
at the hands of white Americans.

Despite repeated reports about the cramped, filthy, and unhealthy living conditions in Chinatown, city officials did little to ameliorate them,

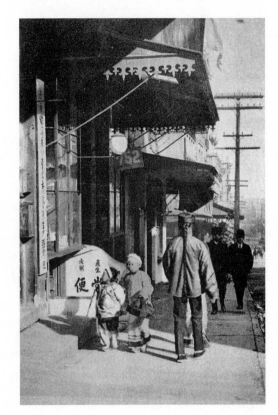

*Many native-born San Franciscans found Chinatown to be simultaneously foreign, frightening, repugnant, fascinating, and exotic.*

choosing instead to blame the immigrants themselves. Indeed, it took the Great Earthquake of 1906, which destroyed much of San Francisco, including the rickety buildings that constituted Chinatown, to inspire rebuilding the area and improving living conditions. But even these attempts at urban renewal were seriously marred, if not subverted, by equal doses of racial hatred against the Chinese, profiteering among slumlords, and municipal graft.[20]

At five o'clock on the morning of March 7, 1900, less than twenty-four hours after Drs. Wilson, O'Brien, and Kellogg announced their tentative diagnosis that bubonic plague had made an appearance in San Francisco (and days before it was confirmed by laboratory tests), the health department rolled out a full-scale quarantine of the Chinese district. This early hour was the usual time that Chinatown's denizens started out for their jobs as merchants, domestics in the homes of rich San Franciscans and in hotels, and laundry or restaurant workers.

As they attempted to leave their neighborhood, the Chinese were shocked to find a battalion of armed policemen vigorously defending against all egress along their neighborhood's boundaries: Broadway on the north, Kearney Street on the east, California Street on the south, and Stockton Street on the west.[21] But because no clear explanation of the public health emergency was offered to the Chinese that morning and a series of gang wars among the Chinese "highbinders" had erupted recently, many residents wondered if the blockade was the city's retribution for criminal behavior in the Chinese quarter. Many law-abiding Chinese were frightened by this possibility since under the hastily drawn quarantine the policemen were now stationed outside the district, and the thought of no rule of law was of far more concern to them than the yet-to-be communicated plague.[22] Others simply worried about how they would earn their daily living if they were prevented from leaving Chinatown for work.[23]

By 8 a.m., the mood in Chinatown was feverish. A team of health inspectors wearing surgical masks and rubber aprons descended and began a house-to-house search of the labyrinth of tenements and the neighborhood's 35,000-plus residents. The mission was to track down every step Chick Gin might have taken during his last weeks and to ascertain if any of his contacts were ill. They were also charged with finding anyone with a suspicious illness who may have had a coincident interaction with the plague.

Accompanied by armed policemen, the San Francisco public health doctors sought out a few leaders of the Chinese community such as Ho Yow, the Chinese consul general, and members of the Chinese Six (or Consolidated) Companies Benevolent Association in order to enlist their help in addressing the crisis. While the Chinese community of San Francisco comprised a large group of many classes, social groups, divisions, and interests, these leaders acted as their representatives and dealt with the city police and health departments throughout the epidemic.

Initially, the Chinese leaders cooperated with the health department's efforts in the hope that Chick Gin was misdiagnosed and the storm would pass quickly. They began these efforts by assisting the health department in writing a circular that explained Chick Gin's suspicious death, the rationale behind the quarantine, and the importance of cooperating with the health department. By the end of the day, large yellow plague placards describing the crisis were posted on telephone poles and kiosks and in storefront windows all over the district. The outraged Chinatown residents, however, found such explanatory attempts to be too little and too late. The following morning, the headline of the March 8 issue of the Chinese-American newspaper, *Chung Sai Yat Po,* declared: "Blockade is a Violation of Law."[24] Only a day later, when interviewed by the *San Francisco Examiner,* Chinese consul general Ho Yow complained about the unfair treatment of his countrymen at the hands of the health department. Doubting both the doctors' diagnosis of plague in Chick Gin and the rationale of the Chinatown quarantine, Ho Yow declared his intention to obtain a federal court injunction against the health board's actions as soon as possible.[25]

The quarantine ropes that wound around the Chinese quarter quickly came to signify something far stronger than braided hemp; they represented, in essence, the social, political, and cultural lines drawn between the Chinese immigrants and the native-born American community. On one side, the Chinese residents protested the unfair treatment, the infringement of civil liberties and the ability to earn a living, and the veracity of the diagnosis itself. Across the rope line, but in possession of a great deal more power, were the San Franciscans who angrily accused the Chinese of importing the Black Death to their fair city and requested an even more stringent quarantine.[26] Perhaps no one made this point more clearly than the mayor of San Francisco, James Phelan: "They are fortunate, with the unclean habits of their coolies and their filthy hovels, to remain within the corporate limits of any American city. In an economic sense their presence has been, and is, a great injury to the working classes, and in a sanitary sense they are a constant menace to the public health."[27]

Oddly, on March 9, 1900, the San Francisco Board of Health inexplicably reversed its quarantine of Chinatown. As health officer A. P. O'Brien explained, "We raised the blockade because the general clamor had become too great to ignore and we desired to injure no more people than was absolutely necessary."[28] One can imagine, then, the confusion and panic that arose on the afternoon of March 11 when an ebullient and somewhat condescending Dr. Kinyoun invited the physicians who constituted the San Francisco Board of Health to Angel Island to look through his microscope at the cultures he made from Chick Gin's glands, the experimental animals (one monkey, two rats, and a guinea pig), and the bubonic plague microbes he was able to extract from all of them.

Within twenty-four hours of announcing this discovery, the one issue most San Franciscans seemed to agree upon was that bubonic plague was a Chinese import. As one anonymous longshoreman observed when hearing the news of Chick Gin's positive plague culture: "It makes one feel gurl durned creepy when you see one of them thar Chinamens."[29]

Forced to react to Joseph Kinyoun's laboratory diagnosis of plague but not willing to appear foolish by ordering still another reversal of policy, the San Francisco Health Department intensified its efforts to inspect and disinfect every home and building in the Chinatown district in the weeks that followed.[30] To achieve these goals, it organized a team of 25 physicians, 50 policemen, 75 inspectors, and 4 squads of ambulances to form a plague dragnet in late March. Personal property was confiscated and burned, Chinese-owned businesses were closed without sufficient explanation, and people were thrown out of their homes so that the tenements could be disinfected. Those Chinese residents whom policemen deemed uncooperative were beaten on their heads and bodies with billy clubs. Such a health crusade did little to inspire cooperation among these immigrants.[31]

More troubling, on March 22 three Chinese residents were discovered dead in a ramshackle tenement and the presumed cause was plague. Feeling somewhat vindicated by the daily ridicule heaped upon him in the press, health board president John Williamson declared the city to be "infested" with plague. The best defense, Williamson insisted, was to "drench" Chinatown with disinfectants.[32]

Even after these diagnoses, however, the majority of the residents of Chinatown continued to express their anger and avoid contact or cooperation with the public health doctors.[33] Anyone slightly ill, whatever the cause, hid from view in closets, alleys, and the maze of cellar-tunnels that connected the tenements lining Chinatown's streets. There were even reports of some immigrants hiding in small boats moored in the Bay or escaping the city entirely. All of these behaviors, of course, increased the likelihood of disease spread if, indeed, plague had truly struck San Francisco.

Americans across the nation read the dispatches heralding the San Francisco plague epidemic in their local newspapers and began to worry openly about the possibility of the germ traveling eastward. State health departments and groups of businessmen and merchants around the country demanded a strict quarantine of all people and goods that either originated from or passed through San Francisco. In response,

San Francisco mayor James Phelan and California governor Henry Gage scrambled to assure an anxious nation that the situation was being controlled and urged that the rivers of commerce originating from California not be dammed. As the weeks of April passed and no new cases were reported, these officials' assurances gained merit. It appeared to many that a public health crisis had been avoided thanks to the efforts of the San Francisco Board of Health. However, the public calm was abruptly destroyed between May 11 and 13, when four new deaths occurred in Chinatown, all of them thought to be due to bubonic plague.

Across the continent, Surgeon General Wyman was monitoring these events from his office in Washington. Kept informed both by press reports and by daily telegraphic communication from his assistants, Drs. Joseph Kinyoun and James Gassaway, Wyman decided that he could no longer trust the local authorities to successfully manage the epidemic. It was time, he declared, for the U.S. Marine Hospital Service to seize control of the situation. As of May 15, the Chinatown "plague problem" became a federal case.[34]

A lthough Chinatown had been the epicenter of microbiologic confusion and contention for almost three months, when the federal government decided to become formally involved, a circus of Barnumesque proportions developed. With great fanfare, Surgeon General Wyman assigned Dr. Joseph Kinyoun to be his "one man in supreme control,"[35] but few Californians were terribly excited by this appointment.

A bit of historical context should prove helpful. Today, when a public health crisis strikes, a coordinated team of local, state, and national health agencies tends to prevail, albeit not without some competition and bickering. At the opening of the twentieth century, however, this concerted approach to disease control was only beginning to emerge. Through much of American history, public health was in the domain of municipal or state control. At several points between 1870 and 1920, the federal government made serious attempts to clarify which entity had jurisdiction over protecting a region's public health in terms of quarantine, vaccinations, and more mundane matters such as sewage, water supply, and street cleaning; but none of these attempts was absolute. For example, in 1878, in response to a terrible yellow fever epidemic that swept the South and parts of the eastern seaboard, a federal Quarantine Act created the National Board of Health and empowered it to take control of the quarantine process only *if* and *when* state authorities failed to do so. These two words alone defanged whatever bite the law's authors originally intended.

A decade and a half later, in the aftermath of a cholera epidemic in 1892 blamed on newly arrived Russian Jewish immigrants, the National Quarantine Act of 1893 was signed into law by outgoing president Benjamin Harrison. This law set up a series of quarantine procedures and public health regulations for inspecting newcomers for infectious diseases that were to be administered by the Marine Hospital Service *in cooperation* with the state and local health departments. Yet the actual spirit of cooperation continued to vary from place to place and crisis to crisis for years to come.[36]

As the scientific understanding of infectious diseases evolved in the early decades of the twentieth century, both physicians and the American public began to appreciate how germs traveled across city, county, state, and even national lines. The forces of rapid transportation, urbanization, industrialization, and mass immigration that characterized this period demanded a centralized administration of public health issues. As a consequence, the local control of public health was gradually surrendered to a national approach. Nevertheless, whenever the federal officials descended on a city for reasons of public health, there was (and is) local grumbling and, at times, outright obstruction.[37]

Internecine politics and battles aside, the discovery of new plague cases forced the San Francisco Health Department to submit to a four-pronged plan of attack imposed by the U.S. Marine Hospital Service. Specifically, Surgeon General Wyman ordered a complete cordon sanitaire around Chinatown, mass inoculations with the experimental Haffkine plague vaccine, intensive disinfection efforts of every Chinese and Japanese dwelling in the region, and the prevention of all Chinese and Japanese residents, but not others, from traveling outside San Francisco.[38]

Within hours of receiving Wyman's telegraphed orders from Washington, a ring of armed policemen was reinstated around the periphery of Chinatown. This human barrier was curiously perforated by a policy whereby white, native-born American merchants could enter and exit Chinatown freely. Similarly, if a white business was directly across the street from a Chinese one, the quarantine border was gerrymandered so that the white business or tenement was excluded from the area of enforced isolation. The double standard, of course, was counterintuitive to what was scientifically understood about plague at the time; after all, if one of these white merchants had been infected, the disease would have spread just as easily as if a Chinese resident contracted it. Some public health physicians dismissed these complaints with convoluted medical explanations that plague primarily struck those who ate diets rich in grains, such as rice, as opposed to the more American diet that featured plenty of meat. Understandably, the Chinese residents of San Francisco vigorously objected to the edict's duplicity, no matter how important the public official who ordered it or its pseudo-scientific rationale. As with the first quarantine effort, the second attempt continued to be imposed by the heavy hand of its enforcers: the health officials and the police department who paraded through the twelve-block neighborhood evicted Chinese residents, burned personal property, and brutally beat those who did not cooperate.[39]

Although not as politically powerful as it was in the late nineteenth century, the Six Companies Benevolent Association represented their Chinese brethren as best they could, particularly when those needs coincided with the commercial interests of the community's wealthiest members. The benevolent society devoted its resources toward a wide variety of efforts to educate, employ, and help Chinese newcomers adjust to life in America, as well as to provide health care and burial assistance.[40]

Along with the Chinese counsel general's office, the Six Companies worked tirelessly on behalf of the residents of Chinatown during the epidemic. Eager to simultaneously help their constituents and facilitate the city's efforts to eradicate the plague, they walked a narrow and unstable bridge stretched across a canyon of easily aroused anger. The Six Companies' stance during the first quarantine in March was essentially cooperative. But as May passed into June and the second quarantine threatened to go on indefinitely, they became far more impatient. For example, on June 1 the benevolent association formally petitioned the city of San Francisco to provide food and financial assistance for the isolated and impoverished Chinese residents. A few native-born Americans echoed these requests, including the former U.S. congressman James G. MacGuire: "The Chinese are practically prisoners, and we who are their keepers should see that they do not suffer."[41] Sadly, the Chinese community's pleas failed to inspire Mayor James Phelan to take any action beyond scolding them: "The Six Companies profit by the Chinese in normal times and should provide for them now . . . [the Chinese] suffer from the consequences of their acts, after constant notice, and are not entitled to any consideration of the 'kind proposal.' . . . Let them make Chinatown sanitary, permit inspectors to reveal their side and subject themselves to the laws which govern us all."[42]

The Six Companies and Consul General Ho Yow reprimanded the mayor for the city's insensitive actions, but succeeded only in eliciting more scorn. Most vociferous in blaming the victims for their hunger was William Randolph Hearst, the publisher of the *San Francisco Examiner:* "When Consul-General Ho Yow puts forth another demand in behalf of his countrymen let him remember that they are here on sufferance and that we have grounds for complaint ourselves."[43] Apparently Hearst did not read his own newspaper before sitting down to write his editorial. The food stalemate was settled quietly a day before his column appeared. A group of businessmen led by the German Jewish immigrant Levi Strauss, who is best recalled as the founder of the company that made blue jeans a staple of the world's wardrobe, raised the necessary funds to provide food for the quarantined Chinese.[44]

Food alone did not calm the rising tide of mistrust and anger in Chinatown. On the morning of June 1, a group of Chinese men surrounded a health official inspecting a neighborhood well and accused him of poisoning their water supply. Armed with bricks and bats, the men shouted, "Kill him! Beat him! Make him eat his own poison!" Fortunately for the health inspector, a policeman arrived on the scene who was well known for treating the Chinese with fairness and respect. The two escaped with their lives, but both immediately demanded to be reassigned to a safer district. As Consul General Ho Yow observed: "So great is the fear of poisoning among the Chinese that many of our people would prefer to starve rather than eat food which has passed through the hands of the 'white doctors.' "[45]

Who should be allowed to examine and treat the ill was another point of contention among the Chinatown residents, as was the veracity of the plague diagnoses. Many Chinese residents simply refused to believe the San Francisco or federal doctors' claims that *Yersinia* had descended upon their neighborhood. These beliefs were not entirely unjustified. During the first days of June, of the eight "plague diagnoses" discovered in Chinatown since Chick Gin's death, four were subsequently changed to other causes.[46] The Six Companies requested that the local and federal authorities allow Chinese physicians to accompany the health inspectors charged with examining potential plague patients. The health department denied all such requests.[47]

The civil unrest only intensified on June 5 when the health team announced, at the insistence of Surgeon General Wyman, its plans to move approximately 1,000 to 1,500 Chinese residents en masse to a detention camp on either Angel Island or Mission Rock. In fact, the surgeon general telegraphed his assistants in San Francisco on a daily basis, urging them to convince the local authorities to isolate the Chinese in a more definitive manner rather than simply cordoning off Chinatown. After learning about these efforts, Consul General Ho Yow warned that they would inspire only further mob violence: "My people will never submit to such a detention camp scheme . . . the feeling among the Chinese is such that they would prefer to risk their lives rather than be compelled to remain in the power of American physicians for an indefinite period."[48]

Perhaps the most incendiary attempt to halt the plague's spread was Surgeon General Wyman's order to inoculate every Chinese and Japanese resident of San Francisco with the Haffkine plague prophylactic vaccine. Developed three years earlier by the Swiss bacteriologist Waldemar Haffkine in response to an epidemic raging in India, the Haffkine vaccine was a popular if not well-proven preventive agent.[49] Given that no medication yet existed that was assured to successfully cure bubonic plague, one can begin to understand the excitement generated in the medical community about what today would be called an experimental product. Recently, several historians have criticized the use of the vaccine in 1900 because of its propensity for a number of nasty side effects, ranging from a few days of fever, local swelling and pain at the injection site, and generalized achiness to, in a few cases, death. Such critiques benefit significantly from the comfort of hindsight and beg the obvious question: when threatened with bubonic plague in Chinatown of 1900, what other medical measures did the health officers have to halt it?

The Chinese residents were well acquainted with the vaccine's dangerous side effects because they were widely reported and discussed in the Chinese immigrant press. For example, when the Haffkine vaccine was used in India in 1897, fourteen deaths in one Punjab village alone were ascribed to the vaccine, although Dr. Haffkine later explained these fatalities as the result of a contaminated batch. More problematic was the fact that some vaccinated people still contracted plague. Thus, when the vaccination corps came through Chinatown in mid to late May armed with their hypodermics, they found few takers.[50]

That same day, the Chinese Six Companies and Consul General Ho Yow sent a telegram to his brother-in-law, the Chinese minister in Washington, Wu Ting-fang, reporting the forcible inoculations by the health officers and the intense Chinese resistance: "all Chinese object; would rather go back to China than subject." The telegram also urged the Chinese minister to do something to halt the efforts with the stern warning: "If they inoculate by force there might be trouble and bloodshed and may lead to serious complications." Ho Yow further observed, in an interview with the *Sacramento Record-Union,* that many of the Chinese who had been inoculated with the Haffkine vaccine, including his own clerk, were now deathly ill.[51]

In early June, hoping that a successful result would encourage others to follow suit, a public health physician named Frank Fitzgibbon convinced a Chinese merchant named Quong Chung to publicly submit to the vaccine. While Quong Chung experienced no detrimental effects from the Haffkine vaccine itself, he did inspire violent enmity among his neighbors. A throng of Chinese men armed with bricks and bats made their way to Quong Chung's grocery store in Portsmouth Square with the intention of beating him senseless. Alerted to the vigilantes' pending approach, Quong Chung fled and went into hiding. The band of angry Chinese satisfied their blood lust by looting his grocery store and burning it to the ground.[52] A few days later, Consul General Ho Yow discussed the event in his daily press conference and warned of worse actions to come if the health officials did not treat his people with respect: "The Chinese are not a warlike people but when driven to it they will fight furiously. They are cornered like rats now. It is well to be careful."[53]

Ho Yow's warnings were ignored, and new forms of civil unrest in Chinatown erupted daily. Many Chinese residents continued to hide from the authorities or escape the quarantine boundaries, prompting an order to seal off Chinatown with a tall wooden fence topped with barbed wire. White Americans justified the harsh public health restrictions with the explanation that the Chinese were crafty, deceitful, and contemptuous of the health department's efforts to combat the plague. In short, those elaborating public health policies and those who approved of them concluded that all the Chinese residents were potential vectors of disease. Few San Franciscans expressed this antipathy more clearly than a police sergeant named Joe Mahoney. Each morning, during the early days of June, Sergeant Mahoney ordered his squads: "Go at 'em with your clubs, boys."[54]

What finally ended the quarantine, however, was neither an economic sanction nor a public health measure. It was a series of court-ordered injunctions. Despite the Chinese community's separation from mainstream American society on so many levels, they organized and put their faith in the American system of fair play and justice. Between 1880 and 1900 many Chinese immigrants became quite adept at using the federal courts to challenge discriminatory laws and practices on the basis of the Fourteenth Amendment of the U.S. Constitution. In 1900 the Six Companies retained the most prominent attorneys they could find on behalf of a merchant named Wong Wai, who refused compulsory inoculation with the "experimental" Haffkine vaccine and wanted to leave California, but could not under Wyman's rules and Kinyoun's guard. A few weeks later these lawyers argued on behalf of a merchant named Jew Ho who maintained that the arbitrary and discriminatory nature of the plague quarantine was unreasonable. The same U.S. district judge, William Morrow, heard both cases. Although he had a reputation for expressing his anti-Chinese sentiments in public, by early June, Judge Morrow ruled in favor of the Chinese community in both cases, calling into question the very existence of plague in California and the racially discriminatory measures of the health officials. Some have retrospectively questioned Morrow's motives because he was a former three-term Republican congressman who may have wanted to embarrass the Democrat-dominated municipal and state governments responsible for the quarantine efforts. But Morrow's decision did far more than score political points; it set a legal precedent that limited the government's ability to violate a citizen's rights in the name of public health or to enforce compulsory inoculations with untested products.[55]

In direct disobedience of Morrow's judgments and in the face of numerous complaints about his conduct to both Surgeon General Wyman and President William McKinley, Dr. Joseph Kinyoun made a few more pitiful and vituperative attempts at resurrecting the quarantine against the Chinese. On June 17, Dr. Kinyoun again tried to prevent Wong Wai from leaving San Francisco on the grounds that the immigrant might prove to be a carrier of plague. Wong Wai and his lawyers retaliated by petitioning Judge Morrow to hold Kinyoun in contempt of court. At the month's end, after several court hearings and numerous lurid headlines in the daily newspapers, Kinyoun retreated with his tail between his legs. The Chinese-American newspaper *Chung Sai Yat Po* celebrated this victory by publishing a bold front-page cartoon depicting a Chinese man injecting a large hypodermic syringe loaded with Haffkine vaccine into the skull of a defeated Dr. Kinyoun.[56] Kinyoun emerged from the plague episode bitter and angry. He was subsequently relieved of his duties at Angel Island on April 6, 1901, and transferred to Detroit, an outpost many considered the Siberia of the U.S. Marine Health Service. A year later he resigned from the service.[57]

Predictably, the raucous, dirty, noisy, overcrowded, and decidedly unhygienic life that characterized Chinatown before the visitation of plague resumed in mid-June as the health inspectors "folded their tents and retreated in good order while a horde of Chinese poured through the lines like the advance guard of a relief column." There were, of course, calls to continue the massive cleanup efforts of Chinatown and even to move the neighborhood to another part of San Francisco with an eye toward creating better living conditions for the Chinese. But these good intentions quickly faded with the waning of the plague epidemic.[58]

Sporadic cases of plague were discovered throughout the summer and fall of 1900. Most alarming, at least to the native-born American population of San Francisco, was the first white plague victim discovered in August. In January 1901, U.S. Secretary of the Treasury Lyman J. Gage, who oversaw both the Marine Hospital Service and the Immigration Bureau, commissioned three nationally prominent plague experts to investigate the health conditions in San Francisco. Their report, using the best bacteriological methods then available, confirmed that plague did, in fact, visit San Francisco. The experts explained that the wisest precaution to take against plague's potential return was not to isolate people based on race but, instead, to intensify cleansing and fumigation efforts in any area where plague was found. Between March 1, 1900 and February 29, 1904, 121 cases of plague were diagnosed in San Francisco with 113 resulting in death. Of these deaths, 107 were Chinese, 4 were Japanese, and 2 were white.[59] Alas, this episode hardly brought an end to the all-too-reflexive impulse Americans often have in establishing quar-

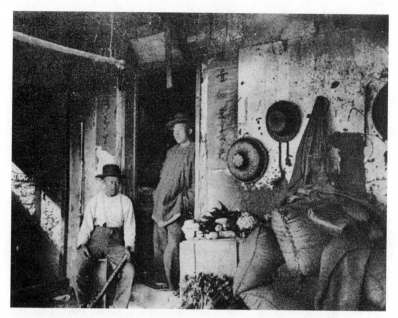

*Once the plague epidemic died down in mid-June 1900, the noisy and decidedly unhygienic life that characterized Chinatown resumed in full force.*

antine or public health policy based on race, ethnicity, or social disenfranchisement.

There does remain one rather strange footnote to the 1900 epidemic that illustrates the plague germ's ability to travel long distances and transcend geographical boundaries. A prominent member of the Bubonic Plague Commission sent to San Francisco in 1901, Professor Frederick Novy, brought some of Chick Gin's plague cultures back to his laboratory at the University of Michigan in Ann Arbor. Chick Gin's plague culture, reproduced in perpetuity, continued to be the benchmark reference point for American scientists studying *Yersinia pestis* for years to come. Several weeks after Novy's return, however, his laboratory assistant, a medical student named Charles B. Hare, who rolled his own Bull Durhams, unknowingly contaminated a cigarette he was about to smoke with some of Chick Gin's plague culture. A few days later he became the first and only plague victim in Ann Arbor and was treated in the "pest house" behind the University of Michigan Hospital.

Twenty-four years later Chick Gin's plague culture anonymously entered the annals of American literature when novelist Sinclair Lewis appropriated this real-life mishap for the climax to his novel *Arrowsmith*. Lewis's collaborator and scientific informant on the novel was a bacteriologist and budding popular science writer named Paul de Kruif. Not coincidentally, de Kruif was Novy's doctoral student in 1916. Readers of this novel will recall that late one night Martin's wife, Leora, assuages her loneliness and fear for her husband's well-being by smoking a cigarette he left behind on his makeshift laboratory bench. Unaware that the housekeeper had accidentally spilled some plague culture on the cigarette, Leora smokes it in an effort to be closer to her absent husband, contracts the pneumonic form of plague, and dies a miserable death before sunrise. Lewis's art did exaggerate real life somewhat; Mr. Hare survived his bout of pneumonic plague and went on to graduate from medical school in 1905, although he died at the age of fifty from a heart disorder believed to be a plague-related complication.[60]

Bubonic plague struck San Francisco once again in 1907 with 160 cases and 78 deaths. In this instance almost all of the victims were white Americans and the public health approach was markedly different. But by this point in history, British epidemiologists in India had worked out the role of rats and fleas in spreading the disease. With excellent rat proofing, extermination, and sanitation methods, the 1907–1908 bubonic plague battle became a war against rats, fleas, and filth as opposed to a crusade against immigrants.

Between 1896 and 1930 there were nearly 30 million cases of plague resulting in 12 million deaths. Since then, bubonic plague has become increasingly better controlled, yet it still manages to appear around the world. For example, a decade ago, in 1994, a serious epidemic occurred in Surat, India, but thanks to medical care, antibiotics, and a vigorous amount of rat catching, the plague germs did not travel far.[61] More recently, in November 2002, a fifty-three-year-old man and his forty-seven-year-old wife from New Mexico were diagnosed with bubonic plague while on vacation in New York City. Both were avid outdoor enthusiasts who often camped out in areas where rodents and fleas were subsequently found to be positive for plague. Fortunately, the couple was quickly isolated and successfully treated with antibiotics. Nevertheless, each year bubonic plague continues to strike some 10 to 20 people in the southwestern and far western United States, and it remains a health threat in the developing world, especially in Asia, Africa, India, and South America, where it kills approximately 3,000 people annually.[62] More ominous have been attempts by several groups and even countries (including the United States) to develop biological warfare techniques that deliver aerosolized plague germs.[63] All of these potential risks recall the conclusions Albert Camus made about *Yersinia*'s indefatigability more than half a century ago:

> [The doctor] knew what those jubilant crowds did not know but could have learned from books: that the plague bacillus never dies or disappears for good; that it can lie dormant for years and years in furniture and linen-chests; that it bides its time in bedrooms, cellars, trunks, and bookshelves; and that perhaps the day would come when, for the bane and enlightening of men, it would rouse up its rats again and send them forth to die in a happy city.[64]

# THREE

# The Rabbi with Trachoma:
# The View from Ellis Island

It was harrowing to see families separated . . . sometimes, if it was a young child who suffered from trachoma, one of the parents had to return to the native country with the rejected member of the family. When they learned of their fate, they were stunned. . . . They had never felt ill. They had never heard the word trachoma. They could see all right, and they had no home to return to. I suffered because I felt so powerless to help these poor people. . . .

— FIORELLO H. LA GUARDIA,
reflecting on his years as a translator for
immigrants at Ellis Island, circa 1907–1910[1]

On the morning of September 23, 1916, the steamship *San Guglielmo* made its way into New York harbor after a storm-tossed voyage that began in Naples two weeks earlier. Among the more than one thousand immigrants aboard the vessel was a thirty-seven-year-old East European rabbi named Chaim Aron Goldenbaum. He was about to complete a long trek of escape from a tiny village in Russia by way of Turkey, Palestine, Egypt, and Italy, when his journey came to an abrupt halt. That year the public health doctors posted along the serpentine inspection lines at Ellis Island examined 298,825 immigrants and almost every one of them was given a clean bill of health. Rabbi Goldenbaum, however, was detained because he was discovered to have trachoma, a contagious disease of the eye that, if untreated, leads to inflammation, scarring, and, for nearly three out of every four victims, blindness.[2]

Between 1897 and 1925 the average annual number of trachoma cases diagnosed at American ports and borders was miniscule, about 1,500, well under one percent of the millions of immigrants who entered the United States during these years. For native-born Americans, alarmed by both the number and types of immigrants then seeking entry, trachoma briefly came to represent the embodiment of germs that traveled. It was a topic widely discussed in best-selling books, newspapers, and popular magazines,[3] and even at school board meetings, where local outbreaks were often blamed on immigrant children and their families.[4] More telling, the doctors who staffed the U.S. Public Health Service (USPHS) declared trachoma to be one of the most serious public health threats facing the nation, and devoted more than 80 percent of the service's financial and human resources to the medical inspection of immigrants at the seaports and borders.[5] For those immigrating, the microbe influenced the experience at almost *every* point along the journey and, if discovered, signaled the end of that journey. And regardless of national origin or Fiorello La Guardia's perception, the disease was widely recognized as distasteful in its appearance, difficult to treat, contagious, and a leading cause of acquired blindness.

Once the major reception depot for millions of immigrants coming to settle in America during the late nineteenth and early twentieth centuries, Ellis Island today serves as a museum of the immigration experience. Since its reopening in 1990, millions of people have taken a ferryboat ride from the tip of Manhattan to the nation's most famous entry point. But, of course, these visits are markedly different from those their forebears may have made only decades earlier.

*In 1916 the U.S. Public Health Service doctors stationed*
*at Ellis Island examined almost 300,000 immigrants. Fewer*
*than one percent of them were rejected for medical reasons.*

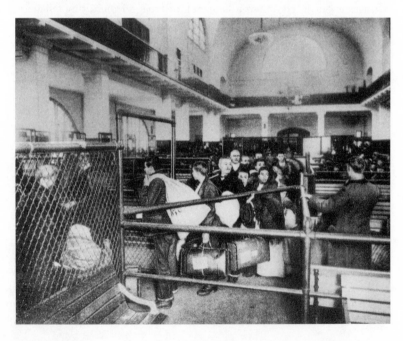

Noise is resoundingly absent at Ellis Island today. When tourists enter its Great Hall they can still see the large American flag hanging on the northern wall and, across the enormous chamber, the tall clerks' desks where thousands of passports were stamped daily, each with an echoing and resounding force. The more inquiring visitor may visit the rooms off to the side where immigrants suspected of having an illness were subjected to intense medical scrutiny, or the chambers where special hearings were held to decide a newcomer's ultimate fate. But so much is missing: the warren of cagelike fences, the rows and rows of benches filled to capacity with immigrants from around the globe, and, of course, the clamorous din.

It is not possible for even the best restoration craftsmen or museum designers to reconstitute the cacophony of voices, a veritable babel in hundreds of different languages and dialects, the smells of thousands of human bodies that had just completed a ten-or-more-day voyage in the bottom of a transoceanic steamship, or the palpable levels of anxiety (if not outright fear) that were once the most pronounced features of the place. It is too quiet, too clean, too vacant for a twenty-first-century visitor to appreciate how bustling, hectic, and for many, harrowing the experience of Ellis Island once was.

Back then, as thousands of newcomers nervously waited each day in the Great Hall, sitting on those hard wooden benches in between a maze of gates and wire fences, they focused primarily on the medical inspection they were all required by law to pass. A team of uniformed U.S. Public Health Service physicians who poked, prodded, thumped, and questioned at seemingly confusing intervals represented the final hurdle that stood between these weary travelers and their new lives. And at the very end of this medical parade was the point where a doctor invaded an immigrant's face and ran a finger across the inner surface of his eyelids to search for evidence of trachoma.

Fiorello La Guardia recalled these diagnoses during his days as a translator on Ellis Island as "heartbreaking scenes" filled with "mental anguish."[6] But with telling and retelling, the role trachoma played in the immigration experience has transmogrified into legend, making historical documentation of the disease and its aftermath quite difficult. Interviews with settled immigrants several decades after their passage range from horrific recollections of the dreaded eye exam to no clear memories at all.[7] In order to move beyond the confusion that the passage of time has added to our recollections of this disease, to see beyond those

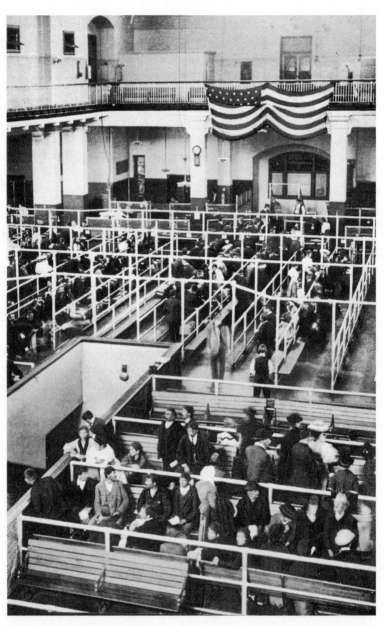

*During its peak years of operation, more than 10,000 immigrants passed through Ellis Island each day.*

stark but famous life-sized photographs of immigrants enduring eye examinations that hang in the Ellis Island Museum today, and to begin to understand these newcomers' intense fear of being diagnosed with trachoma, we will explore the migration pathway of both the microbe itself and, then, one of its many victims during this era, Rabbi Goldenbaum.

At the opening of the twentieth century, physicians had a rather sketchy knowledge about trachoma and their attempts to develop sound public health measures against its ingress were imperfect at best. Today, we accept that the disease is the result of infection with the microbe *Chlamydia trachomatis,* an organism that also causes the sexually transmitted disease chlamydia. But because the microorganism is quite fastidious and particular in its reproductive habits, it is extremely difficult to grow in artificial culture media. Consequently, it was not until

*A Public Health Service physician is flipping up the eyelids of an immigrant with a shoe buttonhook, looking for the telltale signs of trachoma.*

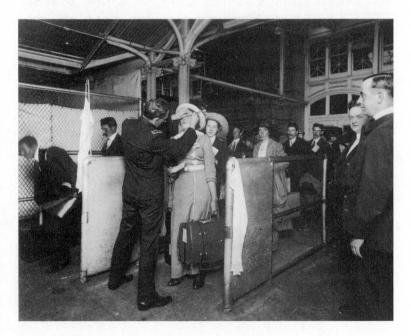

well into the 1940s that microbiologists were able to precisely identify trachoma's exact cause. What was clearly understood by the doctors at Ellis Island and elsewhere in the early twentieth century, however, was that trachoma was extremely contagious.

Trachoma victims wear their stigma on the most prominent part of the face—the eyes. Like the blisters of smallpox or the weeping lesions of leprosy, trachoma seems almost biologically determined to inspire fear among medical inspector and lay public alike, and, in fact, the social response to trachoma has tended to be more dramatic than that to other common, but not necessarily obvious, infections such as tuberculosis. There are, indeed, a variety of distressing signs and symptoms associated with trachoma, but like many diseases it has several distinct stages and, depending on which stage a patient is experiencing, is not always easily recognizable even by the most experienced physician.

Five to twelve days after initial contact with the trachoma germ, most patients merely notice a mild inflammation of the inner eyelids, some tearing, and, perhaps, sensitivity to light. In fact, only about one-third of those infected with trachoma, the most severe cases, suffer from the pus-exuding, granular, beefy-red eyelids that conjure up the disease's most infamous clinical descriptions. After this acute phase, which lasts days to weeks, the patient enters a more indolent phase where chronic and painful inflammation develops—the so-called mixed phase of trachoma. Finally, after months to years without treatment, the reddened and swollen eyelid turns inward; and with every blink, the lashes violently scrape across the cornea, the eye's transparent external surface, setting in motion a vicious cycle of open sores, repeated infections, and, ultimately, destruction of the eye.

For about 75 percent of all those with untreated trachoma, the result is a slow and inexorable loss of vision, much like the closing of a window shade as the eyeball becomes a wasted battleground between the human organism and the microbe. Most shocking to a casual observer are the grotesque blue-white scars that reside where the normal eyes once reigned, making the poor soul afflicted with the disease look almost like an eyeless Greek statue left over from antiquity. In the remaining 25 percent, the body enjoys a Pyrrhic victory of sorts by arresting the spreading infection with varying degrees of healing. But even with this clinical schematic, as one ophthalmologist noted in 1909, "trachoma does not always progress uninterruptedly, there are often intermissions and exacerbations."[8]

Medical textbooks tend to simplify descriptions of disease; the face-to-face confrontation with and diagnosis of an illness is an entirely different matter. Not surprisingly, practicing physicians of this era often disagreed with the public health doctors over individual patients detained for trachoma at Ellis Island. Who was contagious? Who was cured? Who remained a threat to others?[9] To settle these differences, special board of inquiry hearings were held to decide the fate of trachoma-certified immigrants, which could become quite protracted if the immigrant had significant financial and legal resources at his disposal. But the medical opinions of the USPHS physicians, who prognosticated *all* cases of trachoma as contagious, almost always prevailed.[10] Ninety-five percent of the immigrants diagnosed with trachoma at American ports or borders were eventually returned to where they came from.[11] Ellis Island commissioner William Williams explained the matter bluntly in 1910: "It has been demonstrated (what, of course, we already knew) that when our surgeons say that a trachoma case is incurable, they know what they are talking about."[12]

Despite trachoma's well-known association with immigrants, the eye infection was hardly an exclusively imported scourge. It was a common health problem in the United States, especially among poor whites living in the Appalachians, a social group whom one USPHS physician distinguished from the "new immigrants" as "good and honest Anglo Saxon people of the mountains."[13] In a 1911 survey of people living in the highland regions of Kentucky, more than 13 percent of those surveyed suffered from trachoma and many were already partially or totally blind. The Native American population was also profoundly affected by the uncontrollable spread of trachoma, particularly those living on some reservations, where 65 to 95 percent of the residents were found to be afflicted with some stage of the disease.[14] And while Appalachian "hillbillies" and Native Americans had little, if any, contact with immigrants, the broad consensus of medical opinion characterized trachoma as a disease that was imported into the United States chiefly by impoverished Eastern European and Asian immigrants.

Trachoma is a classic contagious disease in that it is easily transmitted by touch. When someone infected with trachoma rubs his own eyes (something most humans do many times a day) and then touches or shakes hands with another, the infected person places the uninfected person at risk for contracting trachoma when the latter rubs his or her eyes.[15] Not surprisingly, trachoma thrives in conditions of poor hygiene and lack of running water. This posed a particular problem for many transoceanic immigrants, given that most steamships were crowded from stem to stern with poor newcomers originating from areas where the disease was known to be common. If one immigrant infected with trachoma was mistakenly allowed to travel in the crowded and often dirty steerage section of a steamship, that person presented a real health risk to the other immigrants in the same compartment.

It was precisely this constellation of risks and beliefs that led Dr. Wyman, the surgeon general of the U.S. Marine Hospital Service, to officially designate trachoma a "dangerous, contagious disease" in 1897. In a memorandum that he circulated to his entire staff, Dr. Wyman declared that the infection was cause for an immigrant's immediate return to the port of origin and "seldom seen except among recent immigrants from the eastern end of the Mediterranean, Polish and Russian Jews, Armenians and others from that locality."[16]

As a result of a series of national immigration laws enacted between 1897 and 1907, an elaborate international system of medical surveillance developed for trachoma and a handful of other contagious diseases, from the deadly cholera to the chronic and annoying favus, ringworm, and other fungal infestations.[17] In fact, the medical inspection of immigrants began long before they sailed into New York harbor or any other American port. The steamship companies, fearing harsh restrictive laws that might reduce the profitable stream of immigrants, hired physicians at each way station along the immigration pathways and at the major seaports to prevent diseased passengers from boarding ships bound for America.

Largely as a result of these medical inspections and the relatively quick passage of most transatlantic steamers during this period (about seven to ten days), it was rare for immigrants suffering from recognizable chronic or mixed trachoma, severe scarring, or blindness to make it out of the European ports. This left only the problem of selecting out those with acute trachoma, a phase that resembles many other forms of irritation to the eye and is difficult to detect without a careful examination of the eyelids. Consequently, the definitive diagnosis of trachoma at Ellis Island was rarely a simple matter and could often be distinguished from more mild eye conditions only with the help of the physician's best friend, "a tincture of time."

Between 1898 and 1905 only those immigrants with watery, red, or inflamed eyes were examined at American immigration stations along both seacoasts. Beginning in 1905, at the urging of several prominent immigration restrictionists, physicians, public officials, and, ultimately, congressional legislation, *all* immigrants seeking entry into the United States were examined for trachoma. Although it is difficult to measure the effect of the more stringent medical inspection regulations and procedures, it must be recalled that the influx of trachoma in the persons of immigrants was never greater than a mere trickle during this period.[18]

Several USPHS physicians offered public explanations of how foreigners posed a clear health threat to American society. One such spokesman was Dr. Taliaferro Clark, who is best remembered today for his role in planning what ultimately became the Tuskegee syphilis study where African-American men were followed for decades to study the natural progression of their sexually transmitted infections but were not given adequate treatment to arrest or cure them.[19] Attributing the nation's trachoma problem to "undesirable" Russian and Polish Jews, southern Italians, and other "new immigrants," Dr. Clark warned that the "unrestricted importation of trachoma is fraught with grave dangers." In a manner that the historian is tempted to label self-serving, Clark urged that strong financial support of the Public Health Service was imperative if the nation hoped to avoid both the economic and physical ills associated with immigration. Not only did trachoma render the immigrant blind and a burden to society, Clark cautioned, the immigrant's germs had the potential to spread to native-born Americans.[20]

Equally bilious when discussing the contagious threat of the huddled masses was Dr. John McMullan, the physician-in-chief at Baltimore's Locust Point Immigration Center from 1911 to 1913. In a widely distributed article he wrote for the *Journal of the American Medical Association* in 1913, McMullan heaped overstatement upon overstatement on the importance of "keeping diseased immigrants out." The good doctor went so far as to insist that a homegrown epidemic of smallpox was preferable to imported cases of trachoma and that the lax immigration laws of the day would result only in the arrival of thousands of "trachoma-infected foreigners."[21]

The same year that McMullan published his trachoma screed, Rabbi Goldenbaum, his wife, and their four children decided to leave their tiny *shtetl* (village). At the time there were several pathways out of the Russian Pale of Settlement, but they can be briefly summarized by two major routes: across the border to Germany or Austria-Hungary and then leaving Europe at one of the northern seaports such as Hamburg, Antwerp, Le Havre, Rotterdam, or Liverpool; or south through Odessa and the Mediterranean. At many points of these immigration paths, particularly along the Russian border and at the large ports of embarkation, the steamship companies operated emigrant medical inspection stations, staffed by their own physicians, who cooperated with the local authorities. The Goldenbaums, unlike most of their fellow emigrants who left through northern Europe for America, were bound for a new settlement in Palestine called Ahuzzat Bayit (which ultimately became Tel Aviv). They traveled by foot, carrying their possessions in a small cart through the Pale southward to the port of Odessa, and after a brief stay in a cheap lodging house, sailed to Constantinople and then traveled by foot and rail through what is today Turkey and Lebanon, to Palestine. The Goldenbaums underwent at least three medical examinations (at the Russian border, at the port of Odessa, and again in Constantinople) and were all given clean bills of health at each point. By comparison, 3 to 5 percent of the Russian Jews attempting to emigrate out of the Pale during this era did not pass their health inspections, and 85 percent of these medical rejections were because of trachoma or eye problems resembling it.[22]

At the close of the nineteenth century, approximately 5 million Jews lived in the Pale of Settlement, a collection of twenty-five Russian and Polish provinces. This population constituted 94 percent of the Jews living in the Russian Empire at the time. Beginning with the infamous May edict of 1881 and subsequent czarist anti-Semitic persecutions, hundreds of thousands of Jews emigrated each year, mostly for the United States and in smaller numbers to Palestine, Argentina, Canada, and other parts of Europe. After the barbaric Kishinev pogrom in 1903 and its successors over the next few years, not to mention famine, epidemics, revolution, and war, the Jewish exodus from Russia only increased in magnitude.[23]

Throughout these years, physicians documented widespread trachoma among Russian peasants, Jews, and soldiers living in the Pale of Settlement. For example, in Kiev, a town heavily populated by Jews, approximately 250 per thousand patients with eye diseases had trachoma. In other regions in the Pale, as many as 350 per thousand patients with eye diseases suffered from the infection.[24] After a visit to the region in 1907, a Long Island physician named Allen S. Busby reported that "one-half of all the cases of blindness in Poland" were caused by trachoma.[25] And while exact statistics of the incidence of trachoma are difficult to come by, it is safe to state that in this particular environment of poverty, overcrowding, and poor personal hygiene, trachoma was a major public health concern.

Early-twentieth-century Russian medical journals and newspapers consistently identified Jews as the source of the empire's trachoma problem. Such attempts at medical stigmatization were not lost on Russian Jewish physicians who had a great deal of experience in treating and diagnosing the disease. In 1908 the *Evteiskii Medtsinski Golos* (Jewish Medical Voice) solicited the opinions of the "world's leading eye specialists" in order to refute the scientific and medical fallacy of claims that trachoma was a "Jewish disease."[26] One Jewish ophthalmologist named Max Mandlestamm, who practiced in Kiev, dismissed the threat as a bigoted means to "scapegoat" Jews and prevent them from emigrating to America.[27]

Several non-Jewish medical experts of the day also refuted the pseudo-scientific claims that trachoma was a uniquely Jewish-borne disease. Most prominent was the German ophthalmologist Julius Boldt, who explained in his textbook *Trachoma* that while no district in Russia was entirely free of trachoma, the disease was not dependent on nationality or race: "all nationalities and races acquire it if the opportunity presents itself. The Jews who are so severely affected in Galicia suffer extremely rarely in Hungary where civilization (and sanitary standards) is much more advanced."[28]

Understandably, the American Jewish community of the early twentieth century was eager to help their co-religionists escape from the Pale.[29] At the same time, however, they worried about the false perception that they were helping to import diseased immigrants into the United States. To counter such charges, activist groups such as the National Jewish Immigration Committee, the American Jewish Committee, the Jewish Publication Society, and the Immigration Publication Society developed numerous pamphlets in Yiddish and several other languages explaining the medical inspection process and the futility of trying to "fool" the immigration officials.[30] Perhaps best known was an immigrant handbook that went through several printings and translations entitled *What Every Emigrant Should Know*. The booklet was widely distributed in *shtetls* and towns across the Pale under the auspices of the U.S.-based National Council of Jewish Women. Welcoming the able-bodied, hard-working immigrant, the booklet's author, Cecilia

Razovsky, firmly warned against the insane, the poor, the criminal, the ill, and especially the trachomatous, making the journey: "Before you decide to leave your own country and begin a new life in a strange land, Think Hard! Consider Long! Decide Slowly! . . . Be sure to be free of trachoma, because America will not let [the immigrant] enter if he shows a trace of it."[31]

To drive the point home even further, agents of these groups traveled throughout Eastern Europe. Along with advice on the immigration process, they delivered countless health lectures illustrated with colorful broadsheet posters that provided exquisitely detailed information on the many ways one could contract trachoma, ranging from communal use of a hand towel to close physical contact with someone who had the disease, and its myriad physical manifestations. The message behind all of these efforts was both to help healthy Jews to leave Eastern Europe for new, and presumably safer, lives in America and to discourage those who did have the disease from even attempting to emigrate.[32]

When the Goldenbaum family began their migration, they, like most Jews living in the Pale, had woefully inadequate access to medical care of any kind, let alone a physician well versed in diseases of the eye.[33] For the majority of these impoverished Jews, eye care meant an occasional visit by an itinerant oculist who traveled from *shtetl* to *shtetl* fitting those in need with eyeglasses. Consequently, the immigration inspections for trachoma were often the first time these people had their eyes scrutinized for any reason, and many were frightened by the abrupt and painful methods employed by the doctors.[34]

The examination for trachoma begins with a physician everting, or flipping up, a patient's eyelid. He then inspects it visually before coasting his fingertip across its inner surface to feel around for the infection's telltale pebble-like granulations that signify the body's inflammatory response to the germ. There are several ways a doctor can evert a person's eyelids, including a dexterous use of the thumb and forefingers; the use of a flat, thin piece of metal, such as a buttonhook commonly employed to lace up shoes and gloves; or specially designed eyelid-everting forceps.[35] But the task must be accomplished quickly, because the physician rarely has more than a few seconds before a patient simply shuts his eyes and refuses further manipulation. Adding still to the need for speed and dexterity, the average control station physician performed hundreds of these examinations each day on the seemingly endless line of those who wanted to leave Europe and Asia.

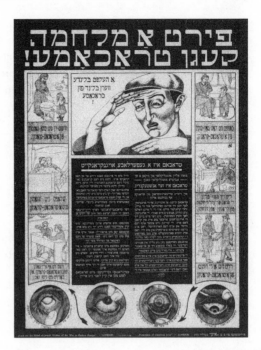

*A broadsheet poster in Yiddish explains in an exquisitely detailed manner the many ways one could contract trachoma—from the communal use of towels to close physical contact—and the many signs and symptoms of the disease.*

Less than a decade before the Goldenbaums left Russia, in 1905, a Jewish American physician and medical author named Maurice Fishberg was sent by the U.S. Immigration Bureau to assess the trachoma problem among emigrants. Traveling to the farthest reaches of the Russian border and along both the southern and northern routes of emigration, Dr. Fishberg observed thousands of Jewish emigrants flooding out of the Pale.[36]

German law prohibited East European emigrants from stopping over in any city of the empire following the 1892 cholera epidemic, which was largely blamed on emigrating Russian Jews.[37] To both prevent the spread of contagious diseases to healthy passengers and German citizens and protect their market share, Dr. Fishberg noted, the German steamship companies' doctors isolated the poorest emigrants (those considered most at risk for diseases such as trachoma) at control stations along the German border. A gendarme took emigrants traveling by third- or fourth-class railway ticket—or those even poorer, on foot—into custody as soon as they crossed the border into Germany.

Upon arrival in the major seaports of Hamburg and Bremen, the poorest emigrants were stripped, chemically disinfected, bathed, and, while still naked, examined by doctors to make sure no condition was hidden. They then remained under medical surveillance in fenced quarantine camps until they boarded ships bound for the United States. Those discovered to have trachoma or other contagious ailments were ordered to return to their native land, and, if necessary, a gendarme forcibly escorted the ill back to the border. And while Dr. Fishberg pointed out several flaws and occasional acts of deception in the process, he concluded that the medical inspections of immigrants at control stations along the Russo-German and Austro-Hungarian borders and again before they left Europe were, by and large, a success from a sanitary standpoint.[38]

Not everyone familiar with these protocols agreed. In 1906 one Springfield, Massachusetts, physician named Benjamin Croft was so astounded by the stories he was hearing from his trachoma patients who had been recently inspected at the Russo-German border that he was compelled to write about them for the *Boston Medical and Surgical Journal:*

> The waiting emigrants were arranged in lines and made to pass a physician who examined eyes by everting the lids. My patient declares that the man in front of him was rejected because of sore eyes, and that his own and his companion's, who was next in line, were examined with the soiled fingers of the physician and that the latter was not provided with any means of cleansing his hands.[39]

Equally troubling, a markedly different standard of care existed for those with financial resources. One practice that American immigration officials often complained about was "the second-class scam." Specifically, only those traveling third or fourth class were subjected to chemical disinfections and the most rigorous medical inspections, while those traveling first or second class were spared these caustic "baths" and given a much more cursory examination. The implicit rationale behind the inspection protocols was that only the poor harbored disease. As a result, all who could afford the price of a first- or second-class ticket bought one.[40]

In seaports from Hamburg to Odessa and beyond, there were travelers' aids, legitimate eye specialists, and, in larger numbers, outright quacks called "runners" who preyed upon the afflicted immigrants of

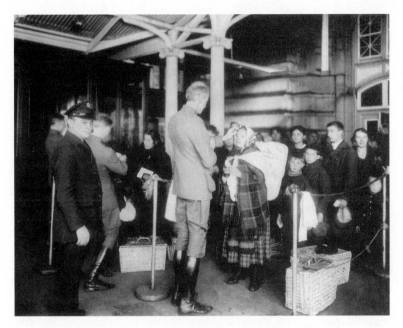

*Many immigrants feared contracting trachoma from
the unwashed hands of the inspecting physicians.*

means. The Yiddish press frequently derided the runners as "trachoma
*shleppern*" (literally, "those who dragged trachoma victims from one
place to another"). These charlatans offered frightened victims false
hopes of rapid cure or, at least, assistance in cosmetic attempts to "fool"
the medical inspectors when reexamined.[41] But even the well-heeled
immigrants could hardly afford more than a few months of the quack
treatments offered by the *shleppern,* not to mention the exorbitant rates
charged for room and board in the port cities, before their money ran out.

As Fiorello La Guardia noted on the other side of the Atlantic, many
families were separated just before embarkation because one member
was discovered to have trachoma. Since most emigrants purchased their
steamship tickets well in advance of their actual departure, a nonrefund-
able expenditure that represented their life's savings, the family member
diagnosed with trachoma was often left behind.[42] Given that there
existed no definitive treatment for the infection, the efficient medical
inspections required before embarking a ship for America, and the

unwillingness of other countries to accept trachoma-stricken refugees, most of those diagnosed with trachoma at European control stations or ports ultimately returned home.

Having successfully fled the Russian Empire, the Goldenbaums found life in Palestine both difficult and disappointing. They were ill equipped to adapt to subsistence farming, and Mrs. Goldenbaum complained that their lodgings were far more primitive than what she was used to as the wife of a rabbi in an East European *shtetl*. Perhaps the issues that weighed most heavily on the rabbi's mind were how he was going to provide for his travel-weary family and whether his oldest, eighteen-year-old son might soon be drafted into the Turkish Army. Consequently, Rabbi Goldenbaum decided to travel once again, this time alone and to the United States, where he heard from acquaintances he might be able to eke out a living and, eventually, send for his wife and children. But in order to obtain passage at Naples, the largest south European seaport, Goldenbaum had to first travel through Egypt.[43] This leg of his journey took almost fourteen months, undoubtedly influenced by the events of what we now call World War I.

As for contracting trachoma during this period, one could not have found a worse region in which to be living or traveling than Palestine and Egypt. In one widely circulated study, British physician Arthur F. MacCallan reported in 1913: "trachoma is generalized throughout Egypt, affecting about 95% of the population."[44] In fact, one of trachoma's best-known aliases at this time was "Egyptian ophthalmia."[45]

Sometime in late July 1916, Rabbi Goldenbaum left Cairo for Port Said, where he boarded a steamer to Naples, a major emigrant seaport that long relied on the advice of U.S. Public Health Service physicians in their medical inspection process. Although USPHS officers were stationed as consultants at several European and Asian ports, in Naples they were granted permission to inspect departing emigrants using the criteria of U.S. immigration laws. The American officials could not bar the passage of a particular emigrant per se, but they could forward a descriptive list of diseased emigrants to both the steamship companies and the USPHS officers stationed at the receiving American port. Given the expense of returning an emigrant and the $100 fine incurred for transporting a diseased passenger, the steamship companies were only too happy to prevent the emigrant in question from making the crossing on their vessels. As a result of these mechanisms, USPHS officials uniformly regarded Naples as the best port in all of Europe for the prevention of diseased aliens boarding ships bound for the United States. During the first decade of the twentieth century, at least 6 percent of all emigrants attempting to leave the Italian port were rejected for some type of contagious disease, about twice the rate at other European ports, and about 75 to 85 percent of these rejections were because of a diagnosis of trachoma.[46]

The majority of immigrants traveling to the United States from Europe during this era made the voyage in the cramped steerage sections of transatlantic steamships. For much of the nineteenth century, these sections were filled to the brim with raw materials such as timber and cotton on the voyages from the New World back to Europe but were essentially empty on the reverse journeys. Capitalizing on the mass exodus of emigration traffic to America that began during the 1880s, the shipping companies outfitted steerage compartments with stacks of iron berths and advertised significantly reduced fares to potential immigrants. It was a journey typically marked by filthy, overcrowded living conditions and pitifully little fresh water or palatable food. Most steerage sections had only a few water closets for all of the passengers on board and a short supply of buckets for vomit and waste. Nevertheless, the steamship lines sold millions of these cheaper tickets to the multitudes that could not afford better accommodations.[47]

Somehow, Goldenbaum saved or raised the necessary capital to purchase a second-class ticket for his passage to America. Unlike the comfortable first-class cabins then available on transatlantic steamships, second-class accommodations were only slightly better than the cramped conditions of steerage. The steamship companies provided bedding and dishes for those traveling in this compartment (as opposed to steerage, where passengers had to bring their own), and furnished these sections with an array of chairs, dining tables, and cheaply partitioned berths.[48]

After federal legislation fortified the medical inspection process once again in 1907, the inspecting physicians were better able to ferret out the majority of those who attempted the "second class scam." But even as late as 1913, one USPHS physician named Alfred C. Reed complained in an article he penned for *Popular Science Monthly* that the chances for "a defective immigrant escaping in the first or second class cabin are far greater than [in] the steerage."[49]

While we can probably assume that when the port physicians examined Rabbi Goldenbaum before leaving Naples he was free of infection, it is impossible to confirm this with absolute certainty. He may have had an incipient case of trachoma before boarding the vessel or he may have contracted the infection during the voyage. When reflecting on his travels through the Middle East and the strict regulations against those discovered to have trachoma, however, Goldenbaum likely considered the second-class ticket a wise investment to make in the event that he did have the disease.

Little is documented about the voyage of the *San Guglielmo*. The 8,341-ton ship owned by the Sicula Americana Line left Naples on September 9, 1916, and was making one of her final voyages to New York. (The ship was wrecked near Loano, Italy, on January 18, 1918.) The fourteen-day journey to America was almost twice as long as the average transatlantic crossing, but it also included brief stops in Messina and Palermo before heading for New York.[50] There were 1,019 passengers, mostly Greek and Italian emigrants, in the steerage and another 93 in the second-class compartment. From other contemporary descriptions of transatlantic immigrant steamship passage during this period, we know that ocean travel was hardly beneficial to ocular health. Wind, salt air, unhygienic living conditions, and sporadic access to clean water for washing often led to irritation of the emigrants' eyes, making them prone to all types of infections, ranging from the benign viral conjunctivitis to the more chronic and debilitating trachoma. The most common explanation for emigrants with red, teary eyes upon arrival in the United States, incidentally, was that many of them were crying—out of fear, excitement, or other emotions experienced during the voyage and just before medical inspection.[51]

The *San Guglielmo* entered New York harbor on the morning of September 23. After a brief inspection at the New York State Quarantine Station, off Staten Island, to search for evidence of cholera, typhus, plague, yellow fever, and smallpox, the ship dropped her anchor in the Lower Bay. There, the USPHS physicians boarded the vessel to examine the second-class passengers and to arrange for the transfer of all the steerage passengers to Ellis Island. In consultation with the ship's surgeon, one Parcelhuis Albino, who had ten years' experience on the Sicula Americana Line, a total of 186 passengers, from both the steerage and the second-class compartments, were earmarked for special inquiry inspections on Ellis Island. Among this group was the five-foot-seven-inch black-haired rabbi.[52]

During the Progressive Era, government bureaucrats heralded Ellis Island as a paragon of the principles of "scientific management."[53] By 1907, the peak year of human traffic flowing through the Great Hall, it was not uncommon for more than ten thousand immigrants to be medically inspected on any given day. Yet the number of doctors who actually performed the herculean task of examining all of these newcomers was shockingly small.

When Ellis Island opened its doors in 1892, there were 6 physicians stationed to inspect the roughly 200,000 immigrants who streamed through that year. After hearing the details of this operation, Dr. Henry Hurd, the superintendent of the Johns Hopkins Hospital, pointedly asked, "How can a physician inspect two thousand persons as they should be in a couple of hours, when it sometimes takes a doctor twice that long to diagnose one patient?"[54] By 1902, the number of examining physicians increased to 8 for over 500,000 arrivals; and in 1905 when almost 900,000 immigrants were processed at Ellis Island, there were 16 medical officers. On the day Rabbi Goldenbaum walked into the Great Hall in the fall of 1916, there were 25 physicians and 4 inspection lines running simultaneously. Even with this increase in medical personnel, on busy days immigrants often waited as long as forty-eight hours for their final inspection.[55]

Nevertheless, almost every physician who worked for the U.S. Public Health Service swore by this "systematic and intelligent" protocol.[56] Many historians, and not a few practicing physicians, have retrospectively questioned the humane impulses of those who designed "the Line." But given the paucity of imported epidemics during these years, it remains hard to challenge its efficiency in quickly identifying which immigrants were ill and a danger to others.

The process essentially began soon after the immigrants walked onto the island. They were told to carry their bags into the main building and up a long flight of steps. Those who had to stop in the middle of this path, clutching their chests in pain or short of breath, were pulled aside to be inspected for evidence of chronic heart disease, such as atherosclerosis or damage from a long-ago bout with rheumatic fever, or lung problems. This was hardly the end of their endurance tests. As the immigrants carried their suitcases and trunks across the Great Hall, another physician was watching them closely to detect abnormalities in posture, muscular weakness, or a lame gait. After this, immigrants were asked to turn at right angles so a physician could inspect both sides of their face for sym-

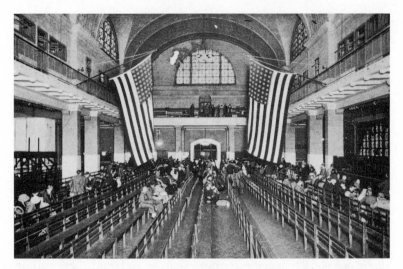

*On particularly busy days, immigrants often waited as long as forty-eight hours before being inspected and processed through Ellis Island.*

metry or defects, and the neck for evidence of goiter. At other points, their vision was tested, a stethoscope was placed on their chests to listen to their hearts and lungs, and, later still, their nails, skin, and scalp were inspected for evidence of fungal infections. Those who appeared "odd" or who could not follow directions were scrutinized for mental acuity or evidence of psychiatric disabilities. The final portion of this assembly line process was dedicated to the doctor's inspection of the eyelids and eyes for evidence of trachoma.

Several descriptions of the trachoma examinations published in official government reports as well as popular magazine articles document scrupulous attention paid to sanitary techniques. Indeed, these accounts present the USPHS doctors as practitioners of the most modern scientific methods of the day for preventing the incursion of disease.[57] Yet there were occasional eyewitness accounts of a decidedly unhygienic "Line."[58] One of the most prominent critics of the Ellis Island medical examinations was President Theodore Roosevelt. Long sensitive to the needs and, more acutely, the political clout of immigrants who became naturalized citizens, Roosevelt visited Ellis Island several times during his presidency. After one such visit in 1906, TR wrote his secretary of commerce and labor, Victor H. Metcalf: "I was struck by the way in which the doctors made the [trachoma] examinations with dirty hands and with no pretense to clean their instruments, so that it would seem to me that these examinations as conducted would themselves be a fruitful source of carrying infection from diseased to healthy people."[59]

Although numerous public health reports stressed the point that physicians sterilized their hands and instruments between immigrant examinations, very few of the extant archival photographs documenting the examination process support such a claim.[60] By 1916, most of the physicians routinely cleaned their hands and instruments, whether buttonhooks or forceps, with the disinfectant Lysol between examining patients. But we also know that some USPHS physicians still used the thumb and forefinger technique, with or without wearing surgical gloves, until at least 1923.[61] Regardless of technique, many immigrants worried about the possibility of contracting trachoma, literally, at the

*Theodore Roosevelt visited Ellis Island many times during his presidency and was struck by the failure of the inspecting physicians to wash their hands or instruments in between examining immigrants for trachoma.*

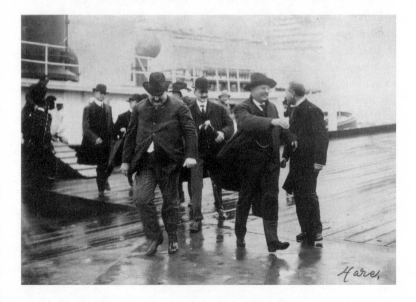

hands of an inspecting physician at Ellis Island; and when considering the massive volume and speed with which these examinations were performed, it is possible that on occasion, hands or instruments were not properly disinfected.

Rabbi Goldenbaum's tour through Ellis Island began late in the afternoon on the day of his arrival. Although he quickly passed through most of his medical inspection, soon enough the rabbi came to the point in the Line where his eyes were to be examined. The physician on duty everted Goldenbaum's eyelids, as he must have done thousands of times a day, but slowed his tactile examination when his fingertip sensed a patch of tiny raised bumps. The physician consulted a few of his colleagues working on the Line that day to confirm his tentative diagnosis, as was the standard practice on Ellis Island. All of the doctors agreed that while mild and recent in origin, the rabbi was probably suffering from trachoma. The inspecting physician then picked up a broad blue piece of chalk and scrawled the letter "T" (for trachoma) on the rabbi's overcoat. Goldenbaum was one of 920 immigrants coming to America in 1916 diagnosed with trachoma.

No mere graffito, the chalk mark relegated the rabbi to a five-day stay at the Contagious Disease Hospital. There, self-limited cases of viral conjunctivitis or simply inflamed eyes, the symptoms of which typically resolve in a few days, could be more easily distinguished from those of trachoma. After this period of observation, those diagnosed with "untreatable" trachoma were sent back to their port of origin on the same steamship line on which they arrived. Depending on the health of the immigrant and the schedule of the steamship lines, this could take another few days to weeks.

For those with early stage trachoma infections who remained at the hospital, the course of treatment was protracted and expensive. The average time spent on the trachoma ward at the Ellis Island Hospital was about six months, a striking comparison to all other medical problems treated there, which resulted in an average length of stay of about ten to fifteen days.[62] Understandably, the U.S. government was hesitant to accept many of these chronic cases, as were the local hospitals of New York City, even those that catered to immigrants.[63] As a result, only about one hundred immigrants, those deemed most likely to recover, were treated for trachoma at Ellis Island each year. But before a hospital

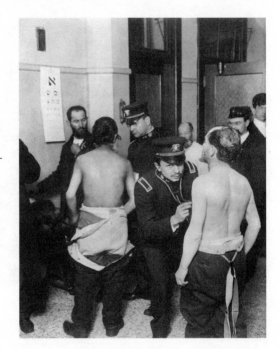

*U.S. Public Health Service doctors examining a group of East European Jewish men at Ellis Island, circa 1916*

admission could be ordered, each immigrant facing debarment appeared before special boards of inquiry held to discuss the merits of his or her case.[64]

The rabbi had three factors working in his favor when the board of inquiry met to discuss his fate on September 28, 1916. First was the early stage of his eye disease. Second, deportation had become less palatable on humanitarian grounds with the onset of war in Europe. Third, the East European Jewish American community was beginning to establish itself within the broader fabric of American society and providing assistance to fellow newcomers.

In New York City, where more than half of all East European Jewish immigrants settled, there were hundreds of synagogues, benevolent organizations, immigrant-run financial institutions and businesses, kosher butchers and restaurants, Yiddish newspapers and magazines, a burgeoning labor movement, and entertainment venues ranging from the famed Yiddish theater to crossover acts in American vaudeville and the legitimate theater, not to mention the social organizations developed

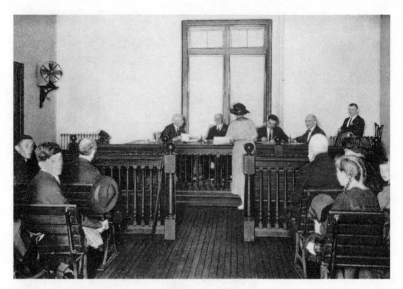

*The Board of Special Inquiry Hearing Room at Ellis Island served as the court of appeals for immigrants who were likely to be rejected.*

by the German Jewish immigrants who had arrived decades earlier and were far more well established in American society.[65] There also existed several immigrant aid societies, such as the Hebrew Immigrant Aid Society (HIAS) founded in 1902, dedicated to improving conditions at Ellis Island and the care and comfort of those immigrants who were detained.[66]

For those who required medical treatment at Ellis Island, immigrant aid societies like HIAS acted as middlemen between the detained immigrant and his family members (if any existed) already settled in the United States. Health care for impoverished Americans and immigrants was sporadic in the early decades of the twentieth century, and what little was offered was largely underwritten by private citizens and philanthropic groups.[67] Immigrant aid society agents contacted an ill newcomer's relatives and urged, cajoled, and at times outright harangued them to make sure all medical costs were paid for, in advance. Such an expense was often a financial drain on the relative, who may have been struggling himself to earn a living. The more distant the relationship, the more often the relative declined to come up with the necessary funds, resulting in the immigrant being sent back to the port of origin.[68]

Another common way for immigrant families to raise money for needy or ill relatives detained at Ellis Island was to organize parties, dinners, and benefit productions of Yiddish plays. In New York City alone, there were more than a dozen professional Yiddish acting troupes, all of which relied upon the *landsmanshaftn* (immigrant social groups) buying blocks of tickets for a meal and an evening of entertainment at reduced rates.[69] On many occasions the plays themselves and the popular songs sung at these events were about the travails of the East European Jewish immigrant.[70]

At his hearing, Goldenbaum was represented by an HIAS agent named Samuel Frommer, who was multilingual and well versed in the international art of the *noodge*.[71] Frommer pledged to the immigration officials that his society was willing to underwrite all expenses related to the rabbi's treatment both on Ellis Island and thereafter. HIAS, a dedicated group with only fledgling financial resources, was rarely so bold in its support efforts. But because of the reverence the Jewish American community still held for their religious leaders and the cultural importance they placed on charitable acts, the agent must have been confident that HIAS would not be alone in the payment of the rabbi's hospital bills. Apparently, the board of inquiry and the Ellis Island doctors agreed with Frommer's presentation and Rabbi Goldenbaum was formally admitted to the trachoma ward of the Ellis Island Contagious Disease Hospital later that day.

The treatment for trachoma employed at Ellis Island in 1916 was, by today's standards of care, brutal. This was not an issue of poor medical care or insensitive treatment; indeed, the Ellis Island doctors probably had as much or more experience with the diagnosis and treatment of trachoma than those at any other medical facility in the world. At this point in history, however, medications reliably capable of vanquishing the infection simply did not exist. The treatment of choice, then, was to facilitate the body's natural attempt to cure itself and, if necessary, surgically remove both the diseased tissue and a wide margin of healthy tissue to prevent further spread and recurrence of the infection.

Initially, the Ellis Island doctors confined Rabbi Goldenbaum to a darkened room where cold compresses were applied to his eyes for an hour at a time at two-hour intervals, four times a day, followed by washing his eyes with antiseptic solutions. Several weeks of this mild therapy, however, failed to clear up the rabbi's trachoma, and his doctors decided to perform a procedure called follicular expression. Goldenbaum was taken to the operating room where his eyelids were everted and painted with a liquid form of cocaine as an anesthetic. Following this, a surgeon used a specially designed roller forceps to express, or squeeze out, the infectious contents of the trachoma granulations and induce a moderate hemorrhage or bruise. The surgeon then performed an operation called scarification where the doctor makes a series of tiny, shallow incisions on the inner surface of the patient's eyelids. As an adjunct to this surgical approach, the doctors treated the rabbi with bluestone, a type of copper sulfate that was rubbed onto the diseased areas. Another procedure the rabbi subsequently endured was called grattage, the vigorous rubbing of the inner eyelids with a steel, toothbrush-like instrument dipped in corrosive chemicals such as bichloride of mercury.[72]

These painful treatments were far from obscure to the immigrant community and even formed the basis for one of the most graphic installments of the illustrious Yiddish writer Sholom Aleichem's last book, *Off for America*. The novel found a huge audience among both Yiddish and American readers only months before Rabbi Goldenbaum was detained at Ellis Island when it was translated into English and serialized in the famed Sunday magazine of Joseph Pulitzer's *New York World* between January and June 1916. With national syndication, approximately five million Americans, not to mention Sholom Aleichem's legion of Yiddish-speaking readers, read these poignant stories.[73]

In the installment published on March 26, 1916, Sholom Aleichem recounts the story of an immigrating family about to leave Antwerp for America. Sadly, the youngest daughter, Goldele, is diagnosed with trachoma and must stay behind. Nearly a year passes, yet poor Goldele remains apart from her parents and siblings. In Antwerp, the little girl lives in a cheap boardinghouse with another trachoma patient and hopeful emigrant named Mrs. Zeitshuk. Both see the same trachoma doctor for regular treatments without much success, but Mrs. Zeitshuk blames Goldele's lack of progress on the little girl's constant crying. Goldele, on the other hand, has an informed explanation for her continued eye problems—germ theory: "[It's] on account of the blue-stone! Every time that

I come to the doctor, he rubs my eyes with the same blue-stone he uses on the other patients. If I could afford to have a blue-stone of my own I would have been cured long ago. . . . Then perhaps I might be able to see my papa and mama."[74]

It is entirely possible that if a particular bluestone was used in succession on several patients with active trachoma, germs might be unwittingly passed from person to person. Current knowledge of *Chlamydia trachomatis* suggests that it could, theoretically, survive on a wet chunk of copper sulfate for several minutes after initial contact. But even if the bluestone was washed and disinfected between uses on different patients, the comment by Goldele (and by extension, Sholom Aleichem) does explain a great deal about both the immigrant community's resistance to bluestone treatments and their understanding about the transmission of trachoma.

Every day during his confinement, the rabbi recited the morning, afternoon, and evening prayers central to the Orthodox practice of Judaism. Between his devotions and treatments, Rabbi Goldenbaum convalesced in bed or, weather permitting, on the hospital's fenced-in porch with a tantalizing view of the Statue of Liberty and the skyscrapers of lower Manhattan. Apparently, Goldenbaum's vision was good enough to write a number of letters from the hospital's library during the winter of 1916–17 on stationery emblazoned in italics with the message: "This letter paper is furnished by the Government, free of charge, to immigrants detained at Ellis Island, New York Harbor, for use in communicating with their relatives or friends." In a tightly scripted Yiddish, Rabbi Goldenbaum detailed his ordeal. His letters record not only a difficult journey but also a medical staff at Ellis Island who did not speak his language or fully understand his cultural and religious sensibilities.[75]

Although several New York City rabbis and some of the Yiddish newspapers made public pleas for Goldenbaum to be, at least, transferred to a hospital where he was guaranteed kosher meals, their requests were declined.[76] But it was not callousness that guided this decision. The Ellis Island doctors simply felt that they were making excellent progress with Goldenbaum's treatment regimen and did not want to disrupt it. For several weeks, the doctors debated among themselves whether to perform another round of surgical procedures on the rabbi's eyes to remove the last vestige of scar tissue. By mid-January 1917, they decided that Goldenbaum's condition was "very favorable," and he was finally released from Ellis Island under the bond of HIAS on January 29. Goldenbaum's first American address was the HIAS boardinghouse at 229–231 East Broadway, in the heart of New York's Lower East Side.

Through the offices of HIAS, Goldenbaum secured a position at a synagogue in Atlanta, Georgia: Congregation Ahavath Achim. Atlanta must have been a strange place indeed for the Yiddish-speaking rabbi.[77] Two years earlier the state of Georgia had shamed itself internationally with the lynching of Leo Frank, a Jewish American factory manager accused of murdering a young woman in his employ.[78] On April 2, 1917, only one week after Goldenbaum's arrival in Atlanta, President Wilson urged the U.S. Congress to declare war on Germany. Two days later, April 4, the Congress was only too happy to comply. If Goldenbaum could have read the April 8 edition of the *Atlanta Constitution,* he most likely would have been alarmed by the front-page headline quoting local U.S. Attorney Hooper Alexander's warning to all immigrants living in Georgia: "Obey the Law! Keep Your Mouth Shut!"[79]

Rabbi Goldenbaum's tenure at Ahavath Achim was a short one, and no record of his stay exists in that institution's archives. Within a few months he left the South to return to New York City, where he earned a living as a Hebrew school teacher, first on the Lower East Side and later in Harlem. Within seven years he was able to raise the funds to send for his family, and they settled in an apartment on West 158th Street. On July 18, 1938, at the dawn of the Holocaust, he was naturalized as a U.S. citizen. Although he had encountered great hardship in his travels and at Ellis Island, unlike most immigrants who were diagnosed with trachoma, Goldenbaum was cured of a potentially blinding disease under the care of government physicians, allowing him to begin a new life in the United States.

A century ago trachoma factored into almost every immigrant's calculus of migration. Today, most Americans spend little, if any, time contemplating its ravages. Those who do visit the Ellis Island Immigration Museum might think about the eye infection briefly if a tour guide explicitly mentions it. But it is not likely to make all that significant or lasting an impression: they grimace, shake their heads, and move on to purchase postcards and souvenirs and catch the boat ride back to Manhattan. Fortunately, while one-half to two-thirds of the museum visitors' parents or grandparents once passed through Ellis Island as frightened, trachoma-dreading newcomers, the disease has ceased to be a threat for Americans. It now seems a quaint relic, an old-fashioned and vanquished problem too often confused with the similar-sounding but entirely different eye disorder glaucoma.

Yet in many parts of the world today, trachoma continues to thrive and remains the leading cause of acquired blindness. Over 6 million people are blind or visually impaired because of it, another 150 million are in desperate need of treatment, and some 540 million people, almost 10 percent of the world's population, are at risk of contracting the infection. Just as a century ago, trachoma disproportionately affects the poor and occurs most frequently in the nations of Africa, Asia, and the Middle East.

Trachoma can be economically devastating in these regions because once a few adults in a small village or town contract the microbe it spreads easily, and, without treatment, many develop repeated infections. Adult women are blinded two to three times more often than adult men, largely because of their primary role in caring for young children, who are the most frequent victims. As older members of a family become debilitated, younger ones take over their roles at the expense of their education and the cycle of poverty continues, unbroken, held together by the microscopic organism *Chlamydia trachomatis.* Each year the microbe is estimated to cost more than $5 billion in lost productivity.[80]

Today, for those with access to medical care and medication, trachoma can be treated safely and effectively with powerful antibiotics. In more severe cases, it can be cured with a simple surgical procedure that takes less than fifteen minutes and is not anywhere near as invasive or debilitating as those performed on Rabbi Goldenbaum. Around the world, philanthropic foundations and pharmaceutical companies under the umbrella of the International Trachoma Initiative are making giant steps to attenuate the disease's influence. In Morocco, for example, these efforts have resulted in a 75 percent reduction of the disease's incidence within a few years. But it could rise again in a heartbeat if these and other public health measures diminish. Hygiene, especially in the form of hand and face washing, adequate access to clean water, and changes in health beliefs and behaviors are critical to managing not just trachoma but almost every major infectious disease the human population is presently staring in the face.[81]

When reporting on epidemic diseases that primarily struck the poor in Upper Silesia in 1848, the famed German pathologist Rudolf Virchow observed: "it is the curse of humanity that it learns to tolerate even the most horrible situations by habituation, that it forgets the most shameful happenings in the daily shame of events."[82] The toleration of horrible situations that affect only the health of others is a phenomenon, sadly, that is still very much with us. While Chaim Goldenbaum and his fellow patients treated on the trachoma ward of the Contagious Disease Hospital on Ellis Island are long gone, the microbe that afflicted them continues to thrive and rob millions of their sense of sight. If he could ascend to a Sabbath morning pulpit today, Rabbi Goldenbaum, a great admirer of the Book of Proverbs, might well have offered this clever passage from its pages chiding us to pay closer attention to such public health threats: "Where there is no vision, the people shall perish."[83]

# FOUR

# Lice, Typhus, and Riots
# on the Texas-Mexico Border

Those who witnessed the actions of the Mexican mob at the end of the
bridge will never forget it. Comprised largely of young girls [incensed at the
American quarantine regulations], the mob seemed bent on destroying
anything that came from the American side. As soon as an automobile
would cross the line, the girls would absolutely cover it. The scene
reminded one of bees swarming. The hordes of the feminine mob would
claw and tear at the tops of the car. The glass rear windows of the autos
were torn out, the tops torn to pieces, and parts of the fittings, such as lamps
and horns, were torn away. All of this happened in view of the Mexican military, which had a sufficient force at hand to stop any kind of difficulty. But
the commanders and soldiers seemed in sympathy with the mob. The
impulse was to injure and insult Americans as much as possible without
committing murder.

> —"Auburn Haired Amazon at Santa Fe Street Bridge Leads
> Feminine Outbreak," *El Paso Times,* January 29, 1917[1]

Typhus fever had been brewing in the interior of Mexico for years. But it was the Mexican Revolution of 1910–17 that inspired the U.S. Public Health Service to classify the contagious disease as one of the most serious public health threats along the nation's southern border. As the revolution displaced thousands from their homes and villages, Mexicans fled their country in droves. And Americans following the situation from the other side of the border, especially in Texas, grew increasingly concerned that typhus was destined to enter the United States in the bodies of Mexican immigrants.

This tense situation exploded early one January morning in 1917 when a group of Mexican women mounted an angry revolt against the immigration officials stationed along the El Paso, Texas–Ciudad Juárez, Mexico, border. They earned their living by day cooking and cleaning in the homes of well-to-do Texans, and each night returned to their homes in Ciudad Juárez. But this particular morning, instead of quietly waiting to cross the border so that they could begin their workdays, the women became enraged over a newly established quarantine against the possible entry of typhus fever. The ironclad measure was established by edict of the surgeon general of the United States. It applied to every Mexican—both immigrants and dayworkers each time they crossed the border into the United States—and included physical examinations, mandatory disinfection of all baggage and personal belongings, and delousing baths with a mixture of kerosene, gasoline, and vinegar.

Most intolerable to the Mexicans was the inherent danger of bathing in flammable and noxious agents like gasoline and kerosene. Only nine

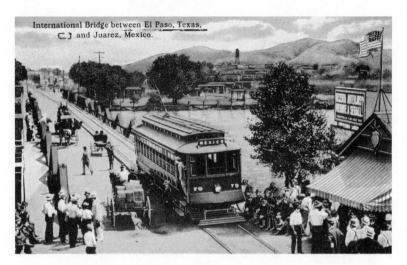

*In 1917 hundreds of Mexicans and Texans crossed the International Bridge every day between El Paso, Texas, and Ciudad Juárez, Mexico.*

months earlier, a group of twenty-six Mexicans incarcerated in the El Paso jail underwent a similar disinfection procedure and, soon after a newly arrived prisoner lit a cigarette, were burned to death. While this practice offended and frightened those who were to be subjected to the baths, its dangerous nature seemed to be all but lost on the Americans ordering them.

Joining the women that January morning were hundreds of angry men, and the protest quickly devolved into a full-scale riot lasting almost two days, including anti-American jeers, bottle-throwing, fistfights, and the overturning of streetcars.[2] As with the germ of typhus fever, resentments among the Mexicans over disrespect and unfair treatment at the hands of U.S. immigration and health officials had been incubating along the border for years.

Rickettsia prowazekii, the microbial agent that causes typhus fever, and its attendant misery have attacked and disrupted just about every society since antiquity. Often confused with the entirely different

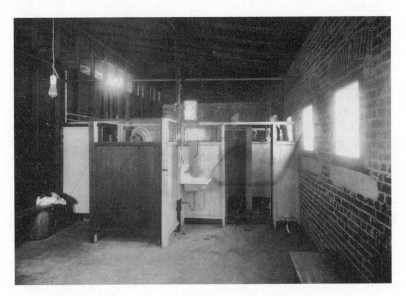

*Beginning on January 27, 1917, all Mexicans, both immigrants and dayworkers, were required to take delousing baths with a mixture of kerosene, gasoline, and vinegar before being allowed to cross the Texas-Mexico border. The Mexicans responded the following morning by rioting at the El Paso Immigration Station.*

typhoid fever—which is actually a gastrointestinal infection caused by a germ called *Salmonella typhi*—typhus fever has rightfully terrified all those acquainted with it. Most likely, it was Hippocrates or one of his students who named the deadly disease *tiphos* to describe its cardinal feature: raging fevers that so disorder one's thoughts the victim appears stuporous, as if staggering about in a haze.[3] More than two millennia later, the noted British physician and typhus expert Sir Charles Murchison eloquently described this foggy state of mind: "[On many occasions] the patient shouts, talks incoherently, and is more or less violent; if not restrained, he will get up and walk around the room, or even throw himself from an open window."[4]

Long associated with filth, starvation, and physical hardship, typhus has been known by many names. Frequent outbreaks among the incarcerated begat the term "jail fever"; among sailors on long ocean voyages, "ship fever"; among starving populations, "hunger fever"; and when it followed in the wake of war and the movement of armies—which it often has across human history—typhus was called "camp fever" or, depending on the specific campaign, "Napoleon's typhus," "Russian fever," and so on.

But while typhus traveled easily from the Old World to the New, it is doubtful that twentieth-century immigrants alone were to blame for its importation. Most likely, the Spanish conquistadors brought the scourge with them in their search for gold and glory, although some have wondered whether the Aztecs and pre-Columbian Indians of Mexico had already experienced typhus before the conquistadors' infamous arrival. One thing is certain, throughout the sixteenth, seventeenth, and eighteenth centuries there were dozens of typhus epidemics in South and Central America which the Spanish settlers referred to as *tifo* or *el tabardillo* (the red cloak). The latter is especially apropos because it not only describes the cloak of fog that descends upon its victim but also the reddish purple spots, the classic rash of typhus fever that covers the body.[5]

By the nineteenth century, typhus was common not only throughout Mexico but in many American locales as well.[6] Indeed, it struck New York City a number of times between 1840 and 1900 and several other eastern cities during the first decades of the twentieth century.[7] Despite this rather prodigious New World pedigree, most Americans considered typhus fever if not exactly a foreign disease, then certainly a disease of foreigners.

For most of its wretched history, as with so many other infectious maladies, the exact transmission and cause of typhus remained an inscrutable mystery. But in 1909 the French bacteriologist Charles Nicolle of the Institut Pasteur in Tunis demonstrated that the human body louse, *Pediculus humanus corporis,* is the germ's favorite means of transportation as it travels from one victim to the next. Professor Nicolle's discovery led to the oft-cited axiom among microbe hunters: "no lice, no typhus." Unlike many infectious diseases, such as tuberculosis (which typically spreads in the air from person to person) or cholera (which is spread by ingesting contaminated water or food), one contracts typhus fever only after a biting encounter with an insect vector, in this case, body lice; although one can easily suffer the annoying infestation of lice without contracting typhus. It all depends, really, on the state of health of the louse that bites you.

The following year, in 1910, the American microbiologist Howard Taylor Ricketts described a new form of bacteria he detected in both the feces of infected body lice and the blood of typhus patients in Mexico City. Alas, Ricketts died of typhus fever before he could confirm his findings. Five years later, in 1916, another bacteriologist, Henrique da Rocha Lima of Brazil, was able to definitively link Ricketts's germ to typhus and he named the microorganism *Rickettsia prowazekii*, commemorating the work of both Howard Ricketts and Bohemian protozoologist Stanislaus von Prowazek, who also succumbed to typhus in the line of scientific duty.[8]

Lice typically flourish in regions where human beings do not have the resources to bathe regularly or change clothing. These many-legged creatures spend most of their day luxuriating in the seams of clothing worn by their human hosts. Such a location constitutes prime real estate in that it allows the interloper a modicum of protection from being swatted away and, because only their legs attach to the fibers of clothing, a great degree of mobility. Cotton underwear is an especially favored site of louse settlement. In fact, many a guidebook of the Mexican provinces during this period urged travelers to wear silk underwear once it was established that the human body louse prefers domestic cotton to the more exotic fabric;[9] and physicians practicing in the American Southwest, such as Arizona physician Francis H. Redewell, routinely advised their patients to purchase silk by the yard, since "lice are loath to crawl over or take up quarters on a person wearing silk."[10]

Soon after taking up residence, these annoying creatures devote their existence to two pursuits, nourishing and reproducing themselves, and it is not long before the mother louse begins to lay five or more eggs a day. Depending on the ambient temperature, these eggs hatch at different intervals. When the weather is warm and the human's body temperature prevails, new offspring called nymphs emerge in about a week. When it is especially cold outside, the miracle of life may take a month or more. And so the process of multiplication continues, leading the famed microbiologist and typhus expert Hans Zinsser to observe: "[The nymph] does not become a sexually mature louse until two or three weeks after emerging from the egg. But then . . . Oh, boy!"[11]

Four, maybe six times a day the body louse and its brethren venture out from the stitched seams they call home to bite their host and consume a favorite meal, human blood. When the body louse riddled with typhus partakes of its meal, rude houseguest that it invariably is, it leaves behind fecal material rich in rickettsia. The human host initially notices an intense itching sensation that demands a vigorous scratch. But with each stroke of the fingernail along the louse bite, microscopic fragments of the rickettsia-laden feces find their way into the bloodstream. Once free of their disgusting vehicle, the rickettsia gain a foothold in their unsuspecting victim and embark upon a dramatic and incendiary torture.

Within days of infection, the typhus victim experiences intense muscle pain, headaches, nausea, thirst, and the onset of high fevers ranging from 104 to 106°F. Such an abrupt change in body temperature makes one feel as if he were beaten about the body and head with a baseball bat. As the rickettsia multiply and travel further and deeper into every avenue and byway of the human body, the patient feels worse. Most people complain of intense dizziness, sleep disturbances, weakness, and exhaustion. Simultaneously, they develop a bizarre body rash, the red cloak of irregular, raised pinkish, purple, and red splotches that look a lot like mulberries. In fact, the "cloak" is really a series of skin hemorrhages or bruises, the physical manifestation of blood leaking out of capillaries and into the soft tissues and skin of the body. This is but one example of how aggressively damaging these microscopic organisms can be.

It is actually the second week of a bout with typhus that is most alarming to those who observe it and, of course, experience it. At this point, the patient enters the delirium phase. The "fog" of typhus is a form of fever-induced madness and is, most likely, a result of the central nervous system's reaction to the inflammation and pathological havoc brought on by the invading rickettsia. The intense, violent battle between life and death finally comes to a close within three weeks. Before the advent of antibiotics, roughly 20 percent of its prey died.

If this morbid procession of symptoms and prognoses were not enough to terrify Americans at the opening of the last century, consider typhus fever's ability to spread, swiftly and angrily, once it strikes a single member of a community. Such rapid travel is a direct result of the body louse's environmental preferences. It seems that lice dislike both the intensely high body temperatures of those who have raging typhus fever and the chilling low ones of patients who die of it. Like Goldilocks of Three Bears fame, whenever the body temperature of their human quarry is anything but "just right," the lice jump off in search of new hosts to infest, thereby further contributing to the spread of typhus. Ironically, the human body louse is even more susceptible to the power of rickettsia than humans, and it almost always sickens and dies within two weeks. But during an epidemic, the typhus-laden lice usually have more than ample opportunity to spread the disease to many more humans before their death knell rings.[12]

Unlike immigrants originating from Europe or Asia, Mexican immigrants traveled by land, often on foot or by rail, to a region many of them still considered to be part of "Old Mexico." The 2,000-mile-long serpentine border that ropes along the southern reaches of California, Arizona, New Mexico, and Texas looks far more imposing on a map than it does in person. Even the Rio Grande, the river that separates much of Texas from Mexico was (and is) a muddy, shallow stream that belies its majestic name. It is an ambiguous boundary that encourages the daily exchange of people.

One observer of life on the border during this period was the famed journalist John Reed. Still a few years away from writing *Ten Days That Shook the World,* his legendary account of the rise of Lenin and the Russian Revolution, Reed was covering the turmoil along the Texas-Mexico border generated by *La Revolución* led by the infamous Pancho Villa. For almost a year Reed followed the clandestine politics and deal-making of the region, rode alongside Villa on horseback, and described the war's devastating impact on the lives of Mexico's poorest citizens, who were often without adequate food, clean water, or decent living conditions. Lice infestations and typhus fever were among the most common health problems that Reed witnessed. Based on his travels, Reed wrote a series of articles that first appeared in *The Metropolitan* magazine beginning in late 1913 and were subsequently published as a book in 1914 under the title *Insurgent Mexico.*

There is some risk in relying too heavily upon John Reed as a historical informant. Walter Lippmann, Reed's college classmate and soon to be one of the most influential journalists of his generation, best described the pitfalls of using Reed as a source. Eight months after the publication of *Insurgent Mexico,* in an article he penned about Reed for *The New Republic,* Lippmann publicly warned readers against trusting everything his former classmate wrote down. "The articles which he sent back from the border were as hot as the Mexican desert. . . . [But Reed] did not judge, he identified himself with the struggle, and gradually what he saw mingled with what he hoped. Wherever his sympathies marched with the facts, Reed was superb . . . where his feeling conflicted with the facts, his vision flickered. . . . He has no detachment, and is proud of it, I think."[13] With that caveat in mind, we must also acknowledge that Reed was touring the region during this period and is someone whose opinions we need to include in this story.

In December 1913, before settling in El Paso, Reed spent a few days in the smaller border town of Presidio, Texas, some two hundred miles away. One night, Reed climbed up to the "flat mud roof of the post office" so that he could get his bearings and begin to understand something about life on "the border." From his perch he surveyed a territory that must have been strange indeed to the Oregon native, Harvard graduate, and raucous denizen of New York City's bohemian Greenwich Village. Looking a mile or more across the "low scrub growing in the sand," beyond the "shallow yellow stream" that was the Rio Grande, all he could see in the moonlight was a distant town "sticking sharply up out of a scorched desert, ringed around with bare savage mountains. One could see the square, gray adobe houses of Ojinaga (Mexico), with here and there the Oriental cupola of an old Spanish church. It was a desolate land, without trees. You expected minarets."[14]

A few days later, the intrepid Reed "waded the river" and "went up into the town" of Ojinaga:

> Hardly a house [had] a roof, and all the walls gaped with cannon shot. . . . Along the main street passed a broken procession of sick, exhausted, starving people, driven from the interior by fear of the approaching rebels, a journey of eight days over the most terrible desert in the world. They were stopped by a hundred soldiers along the street, and robbed of every possession that took the Federals' fancy. Then they passed on to the river and on the American side they had to run the gauntlet of the United States customs and immigration officials and the Army Border Patrol who searched them for arms . . . the inspectors were not very gentle.[15]

Beginning in the 1880s, as American railroad lines plunged deeper and deeper beyond the border into the interior of Mexico, people on both sides began to look at El Paso as a prime location for opportunity and a better life. For Americans, El Paso represented a place free from the problems, failings, and corruption of the older, overcrowded cities along the eastern seaboard. A full-page advertisement taken out by the

El Paso Chamber of Commerce in the March 7, 1914, edition of the *El Paso Herald* exemplifies this optimism. Indeed, Sinclair Lewis's legendary booster George Babbitt could easily have written the advertisement's copy had he settled in Texas rather than in Zenith. In boldface print, the ad noted that in 1910 El Paso was already Texas's fastest-growing city with 39,000 citizens and 7,000 newcomers a year. By 1920, it predicted, the census would surely top 150,000, making El Paso Texas's largest, most modern, and desirable city. From here on out, the chamber of commerce boasted, "the sky was the limit."[16]

For impoverished Mexicans fleeing from harsh conditions as the revolution swept through their villages and towns, El Paso became more than a mere guidepost on the emigration pathway from the interior provinces to the southwestern United States and beyond. It was a destination. Between 1880 and 1929 more than one million Mexicans entered the United States with the intention of resettling. Because of its proximity and economic opportunities, about 50 percent of these immigrants came to Texas, and most came by way of El Paso. By 1920, El Paso had the second largest Mexican population in the United States (after San Antonio) and was the only major southwestern city with more Mexicans than Americans.[17]

Throughout this period El Paso, literally "the Pass," was the economic and industrial hub of the Southwest. Surrounding the city were several rich ore mines and a booming smelting industry. It was also the central marketplace for the cattle and farming industries and, as a result, spawned a network of supportive businesses, services, and workers. Consequently, when sitting down to have a drink in an El Paso tavern, it was not uncommon to find oneself next to a representative (or even a blood relative) of tycoons with names like Guggenheim, Rockefeller, and Hearst—all of whom had substantial economic stakes in the region. Such boozy gatherings inspired John Reed to characterize El Paso as "the Supreme Lodge of the Ancient Order of Conspirators of the World."[18]

El Paso enjoyed both a competitive and symbiotic relationship with its Mexican sister city just across the Rio Grande, Cuidad Juárez. Many Mexicans who earned their living in El Paso resided in Juárez and simply crossed the border every day at the beginning and end of their shifts. At the same time, El Paso civic leaders were eager to push the saloon, gambling, and prostitution trades farther and farther away from their city's center and eventually across the border into Ciudad Juárez. Thus,

American businessmen and traveling salesmen made a reverse crossing of the Rio Grande each night and especially on the weekends to enjoy the notorious red-light district, gambling casinos, and bullfights.

Those Mexicans who did come to El Paso to work, *obreros,* were both welcomed and reviled by their American employers. Needed in just about every local industry and business, the *obreros* were a steady source of cheap and reliable labor that only increased with the Mexican recession of 1906 and especially in the wake of the Mexican Revolution beginning in 1910.[19] Unlike the East Coast, where labor unions and socialist clubs were sprouting with vigor, the organization of workers was not a pressing concern to American employers in Texas and, more broadly, the Southwest. Many industrialists, ranchers, and farmers lobbied their congressmen to bend the immigration laws to exempt Mexicans from restrictions. They even lauded the Mexican's physique as perfect for the working needs of the area. While the East European Jewish tailor, with his rounded shoulders and poor posture, a result of years of bending over a push-pedal sewing machine, might be rejected at Ellis Island because of a diagnosis of "poor physique," the Mexican was considered the perfect stoop laborer because he was "small in size, agile and wiry."[20]

So desired was this plentiful stream of labor that a special dispensation was made in the U.S. Immigration Act of 1917 exempting Mexican workers from many of the harsher restrictions laid down for their European and Asian counterparts, provided they did not permanently settle in the United States. This flexibility of law remains a frequent refrain in the American immigration experience. When a particular group suits our needs, especially to perform arduous labor our own citizens have no desire to do, hard lines become blurred and rules bent.[21]

Early each morning, Mexican men who lived on either side of the border lined El Paso's Second and Santa Fe Streets hoping to be selected by prospective American employers for work in the nearby railroads and construction companies or lifting heavy loads for local businesses. Texan housewives in need of domestic help arrived a bit later to select Mexican women to clean their homes, cook meals, and do laundry. The more fortunate Mexican laborers, almost all men, had steadier jobs in the smelting factories, but for most members of this community, finding work was a daily and uncertain struggle.

As with many American cities of this era, El Paso had a distinct quarter within its municipal boundaries where immigrants settled in great numbers. It was named Chihuahuita, or "Little Chihuahua," because when many of the arriving Mexicans were asked, "Where did you come from?" they often answered, quite literally, "Chihuahua," the Mexican province they just passed through. The ghetto, conveniently located on the edge of the city's business district, was a slum of startling proportions, and life there was hard and dangerous. Mexican residents lived in overcrowded adobe or mud tenements called *jacales* rented to them at exorbitant prices by American slumlords. They had little or no access to clean water, reliable sewage systems, garbage removal, or other critical sanitary amenities. Tuberculosis rates, infant mortality, and other sensitive markers of public health were alarmingly high. Not surprisingly, the district was avoided by most native-born Anglo-Americans, who considered it to be a breeding ground for crime, vice, and disease. Although civic boosters actively publicized their city's salubrious environment, thought by many to improve the health of anyone who settled there from the more disease-ridden metropolises back east, this braggadocio clearly applied only to El Paso's more posh precincts.[22]

Not everyone ignored this glaring problem. In reality, they couldn't. But few of the proposed plans to improve life for the Mexican residents were actually adopted, let alone adequately funded. On a regular basis, concerned citizens appealed to the city government to do something about Chihuahuita. In 1910 a Mexican-born physician named José A. Samaniego beseeched the El Paso City Council to extend sewage lines and garbage removal services to the Mexican district. "These people may be poor," Samaniego pleaded, "but they are human beings entitled to humane treatment. . . . [Chihuahuita would] shame the holes of Calcutta." Within minutes after concluding his impassioned presentation, the city council unanimously rejected the doctor's petition.[23]

That same summer, Grace Franklin, a New York City social worker who moved to Texas to direct the El Paso Women's Charity Association, which organized free baby clinics, milk depots, and summer camps for impoverished Mexican children, made several pleas in the name of the city's Mexican residents. In one speech, she admonished:

[Infectious diseases] may be carried by a horse to the plaza and from the plaza to your table. El Paso must face her problems. She cannot shift the burden with a shrug of her shoulders. The Mexicans are here and every family in El Paso comes in close contact with them, therefore, if El Paso wishes to improve her servant class, she must improve the homes from which this class comes.

Receiving little support in her task, Franklin resigned her post in 1911 to return east. Franklin's successor, Olga Kohlberg, glibly acknowledged her departure with the comment: "[She] was too far advanced for us and impatient of our slower minds."[24]

Throughout this period, frequent editorials in the local newspapers reminded El Pasoans that while the "American" sections of the city enjoyed excellent health, the annual death rate in Chihuahuita was an astounding 32/1,000 residents and the entire city's public health "could not be divorced from the Mexican slums."[25] Despite such urgent proclamations, little was done. Efforts to erect better housing were thwarted by the slumlords who owned the *jacales*. Sewers, garbage removal, and medical care remained scarce services. In El Paso, as in other American communities past and present, blaming the victim was the standard public response.[26]

The U.S. Public Health Service doctors assigned to protect the Texas-Mexico border against diseased immigrants were not nearly as busy as their colleagues in San Francisco, let alone those working at Ellis Island in New York. Up until 1910, the medical inspection process was low key and carried out in a small squat building situated next to the international bridge that spanned the Rio Grande. The examinations consisted of a hurried visual once-over for the most obvious physical manifestations of trachoma, the scaly rash of favus, the dry, hacking cough of tuberculosis, the painless but ugly genital chancre (sore) of syphilis, and the telltale scar of a smallpox vaccination.

The fluid nature of the border, economy, and work culture along the twelve hundred miles from Brownsville to El Paso created a situation of easy crossing that was widely communicated among immigrants from Europe, the Middle East, and Asia. And like the trachoma *shleppern* and other unsavory characters that Rabbi Goldenbaum may have encountered during his circuitous trek out of Europe, there existed a burgeoning cottage industry of quacks and charlatans in Mexican cities and along the border who promised to help those with noticeable eye diseases, skin conditions, and other medical problems—always for a fee, of course—cross safely into the United States.

Between 1897 and 1910 a significant number of Greeks, Syrians, and, to a lesser extent, East Europeans and Asians traveled to Mexico, picked up a bit of Spanish, and pretended to be laboring Mexicans as they

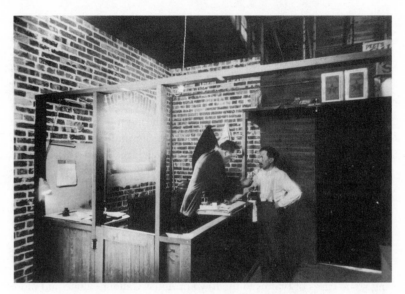

*A doctor examining a Mexican immigrant for signs of*
*trachoma, fungal rashes, tuberculosis, syphilis, and*
*smallpox at the El Paso, Texas, Immigration Station,*
*circa 1915–16*

entered the United States. The ostensible reason for this detour was to avoid scrutiny at the larger immigration reception stations along the eastern seaboard. Officials in Washington became somewhat alarmed over this situation, and in 1906, President Theodore Roosevelt asked the U.S. Bureau of Immigration to look into the matter. In rather short order, an energetic, wiry immigration officer named A. A. Seraphic was given the assignment. In addition to being ambitious and curious, Seraphic was "swarthy and dark complected," enabling him to disguise himself as a Syrian immigrant, affording an unvarnished look at the border inspections.

Seraphic filed a report that garnered attention at the highest levels. Corruption, incompetence, and poor administration, the immigration spy charged in a terse prose, were rampant among immigration officials along the border. At the El Paso border, Seraphic described how the federal government deemed immigrant traffic too small to warrant a full-time public health officer. Instead, the Public Health Service relied upon a per diem physician to inspect those Mexicans, both immigrants and day laborers, entering the United States from Ciudad Juárez. What disturbed Seraphic, not to mention the government officials who read his report, was his discovery that the doctor hired to perform this task was retired, in poor health, and legally blind.[27] But it must also be noted that for most of the years between 1900 and 1930, the reality of imported infection was miniscule. Less than one percent of all Mexican immigrants entering the United States during these decades were barred for medical reasons in general, and the number of immigrants with infectious diseases constituted only a small fraction of that figure.[28]

Several years into the Mexican Revolution, however, health officials did observe a worrisome increase in the incidence of typhus fever in Mexico as well as a mass emigration of Mexicans to the United States. One physician named Carlos Husk, who worked in Mexico for the American Smelting and Refining Company and knew Pancho Villa rather well, presented an alarming report on typhus conditions south of the border to the El Paso Medical Society in January 1916. Documenting 5,000 cases of typhus in the town of Aguas Caliente alone and more than 100,000 cases throughout Mexico, Dr. Husk ominously told his American colleagues: "I think typhus is going to come here."[29]

Husk was hardly the only person announcing the risks of a typhus epidemic traveling north. Throughout the winter and spring of 1916, a cadre of physicians practicing in Texas, Arizona, and New Mexico, the El Paso newspapers, and even national magazines reported on the threat of imported typhus and the need for a strict quarantine along the border.[30] While occasionally voicing concerns about the filthy living conditions in El Paso's Mexican settlements, these physicians were more focused on the troubling fact that more than 65 percent of all Mexicans crossing the border were infested with lice.[31]

Among those most vigilant were the USPHS physicians then assigned to the El Paso–Juárez border: C. C. Pierce and John W. Tappan. Dr. Pierce had just completed a decade-long tour of duty in the Panama Canal Zone, where he did daily battle against yellow fever, bubonic plague, and typhoid fever; Dr. Tappan had only recently settled in El Paso to take a position first with the city health department and then as an assistant surgeon with the Public Health Service. Both these men approached their duties armed with the latest methods in medical science, a zealous devotion to protecting the public's health, and an unhealthy, unabashed antipathy toward their charges. In retrospect, the pressure building up over typhus at the El Paso Immigration Station was almost destined to erupt. When digging through the National Archives records of the El Paso Immigration Station for this period, one cannot help being impressed by the increase in the volume of letters, telegrams, and reports that followed Tappan and Pierce's arrival there. Before this point, the correspondence was limited to annual reports, invoices, and the occasional request for medical supplies. But throughout 1916 and 1917, Surgeon General Rupert Blue could expect almost daily dispatches and reports from the border. The topic, invariably, was the threat of typhus. Although Tappan and Pierce projected a confident air to the El Paso press about their ability to prevent its entry, their letters to the surgeon general document an almost frantic appeal to quickly improve disinfecting facilities and medical personnel.

For example, on March 1, 1916, Dr. Tappan wrote to the surgeon general about the arrival of a train from Mexico City "with five hundred of the dirtiest Mexicans I ever saw." The increased flow of immigrants from typhus-ridden provinces was only the beginning of the problem, Tappan explained, pecking out his correspondence on a government-issued typewriter. Ciudad Juárez, the doctor insisted, was a breeding ground for pestilence: "There were 400 Mexicans [today] on the other side of the river at the Santa Fe bridge looking longingly towards the United States, and they are without provisions, without money, dirty and lousy, waiting to get over here and I have no way of handling them." After pausing in his letter-writing to take an urgent phone call from a medical colleague, Tappan was compelled to add a handwritten post-script: "City health officer reports over the phone just now another case of typhus [in Chihuahuita] which I will go see with him at once and let you know. Doctor, it looks really bad to me here."[32]

Drs. Pierce and Tappan, of course, avidly read the latest medical literature on typhus fever. They well understood Nicolle's dictum "no lice, no typhus," and their approach to preventing an epidemic on American soil was to delouse any Mexican who appeared dirty. Unfortunately, the El Paso facility had only cold water showers for bathing, and showering in steaming hot water is one of the most efficient and safe methods of ridding a person of body lice. But the closest steam shower–disinfecting facility was in Ciudad Juárez, and out of both pride and desire to avoid offending the local Mexican government, the American doctors decided not to make the necessary arrangements to use it. Instead, they began a time-consuming process requesting the necessary funds to build such a facility in El Paso. Both the appropriations process and the actual building of a steam shower–disinfection plant would take another eight months. In the meantime, Pierce and Tappan proposed resorting to the older, and more dangerous, method of delousing: bathing in a mixture of kerosene, gasoline, and vinegar. But before a strict quarantine and mandatory baths for all Mexicans and other foreigners crossing the border could be implemented, the Texas health officers required the permission of the surgeon general, who was still thinking the matter over in Washington.

Drs. Pierce and Tappan were much more successful in persuading the El Paso Health Department to require gasoline baths for those Mexicans admitted to the El Paso Hospital and those incarcerated in the El Paso jail. The mandatory delousing baths became the official policy on February 27, 1916, the same day Morris Buttner, a local health inspector, died of typhus fever. The source of his infection and demise, his colleagues concluded, was his "close contact with Mexican immigrants."[33]

Less than a week later, on March 5, 1916, the local sheriff processed twenty-six new prisoners at the jail, all of them Mexican laborers arrested earlier that day for public disturbances around the saloons of Chihuahuita. At three-thirty that afternoon, the sheriff ordered the Mexicans to strip naked. Under gunpoint, the prisoners, one by one, took a lengthy dip into a large tub that was placed in the center of the jail's communal holding cell and filled to the brim with a mixture of kerosene, gasoline, and vinegar.

About half an hour after this process began, a new prisoner was admitted into the jail cell. His name was H. M. Cross, and he was well known to the El Paso police force as a "hophead." His presumed crime was trafficking narcotics. Still dressed and under the influence, Mr. Cross struck a match to light a cigarette. Even though he was at the far end of the jail cell away from the gasoline tub, there were several naked prisoners milling around him. The air of the cell was thick with the explosive fumes of gasoline evaporating off the deloused prisoners' bodies, and with the mere flash of a match the entire jail caught fire.[34]

The event was referred to in the El Paso papers, and among the Mexican community for years thereafter, as *El Holocausto,* or "the Jail Holocaust." A dispatch in the *San Antonio Express* recorded: "the odor of gasoline mingled with that of human flesh and clothing became so stifling that it was impossible for rescuers to approach the doors to unlock them until oxygen helmets were provided."[35] Despite heroic efforts,

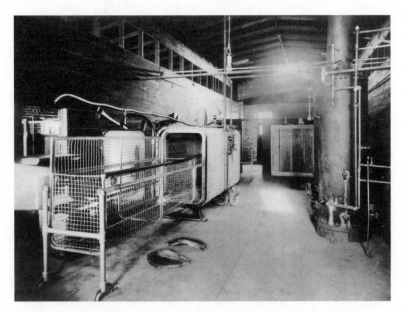

*As a means of halting the spread of typhus into the United States, in 1917 the Public Health Service began disinfecting the clothing and baggage of Mexicans along the Texas-Mexico border.*

including those of a seventeen-year-old woman named Carmen Alonzo, who applied the first-aid lessons she learned on the revolutionary battle-fields of Mexico, at least 26 Mexican prisoners and 2 Americans, Cross and another vagrant named Edward McGowan, burned to death. Another 25 to 30 prisoners were severely burned and injured.

The following day the *San Antonio Express* reported the story of two Mexicans who escaped from the blazing jail and dove into the shallow Rio Grande in search of relief for their burnt skin. From their hospital beds in Ciudad Juárez, the two men recounted to a gaggle of reporters how the El Paso authorities rounded up Mexican men for no good reason, poured gasoline on them, locked them up, and then threw in a lit cigarette to complete the murderous task. All accounts of this horrible event, whether real or exaggerated, garnered great attention among the Mexican residents of Ciudad Juárez, and their response included protests, riots, and mayhem. One American streetcar operator on the El Paso–Juárez line was shot at through his window as he drove the vehicle back from the Juárez racetrack. Fortunately, he survived what turned out to be a superficial bullet wound. American automobiles in the Mexican city were overturned as their drivers fled to get across the border on foot. And anyone or anything else American that remained in Ciudad Juárez over the next few days was attacked by angry Mexican mobs, leading the El Paso police to close the Santa Fe Bridge for three days until the peace was restored.[36]

On March 7 a grand jury was impaneled in El Paso to investigate the event, and its judgments were announced the following day. The police and health officers were not at fault, the grand jury members concluded, the prisoners were. The health authorities were only trying "to prevent the spread of disease from Mexico."[37] The American public health doctors' conclusion from this disaster was that more, not less, rigorous methods of prevention were needed. They felt particularly justified in advocating an even more vigilant guard because of the discovery of a few more typhus cases in Chihuahuita that same week.

Conversely, Mexicans on both sides of the border continued to express anger and distrust. A few days after the conflagration, Pancho Villa and his soldiers made their infamous raid into Columbus, New Mexico, the first successful foreign attack on the mainland of the United States since the War of 1812. Although it may have been a coincidence, the story that circulated among the Mexican community was that Villa was retaliating for *El Holocausto*. Mario Acevedo, a longtime El Paso resident, recalled the event some six decades later:

> I think they were delousing some prisoners and that they were using gasoline to delouse them. And one or two people, from a distance . . . and I should emphasize this: not in an intentional but rather inadvertent manner, someone from a distance struck a match to light a cigarette. You know that the gas in gasoline is extremely dangerous. And it caught aflame. And rumors spread that one or two of the prisoners had been burnt on purpose. And according to the rumors, to the back-alley talk, Villa said: "Now I'll show them how to set people aflame!"[38]

In direct response to the Columbus raid, President Woodrow Wilson ordered General John J. Pershing and five thousand troops to enter Mexico to pursue and capture Villa, a task that proved to be quite difficult.

With the appropriations to build the steam disinfection plants still being debated in Washington, the USPHS doctors in El Paso finally asked permission from the Mexican health authorities to use the Ciudad

Juárez plant. This exercise in international diplomacy was uncomfortable, to say the least. During one of these discussions on the afternoon of June 23, 1916, Juárez health officer Dr. Manuel Nations threatened to close the disinfection plant unless the U.S. government paid him an exorbitant processing fee per immigrant. Tappan heatedly walked out of the negotiation meeting but was unable to acknowledge his part in creating this contentious situation.

That evening, Dr. Tappan wrote an urgent bulletin to Surgeon General Rupert Blue. He was absolutely convinced that the United States was going to be invaded by typhus in the bodies of Mexican dayworkers from Juárez. In this official correspondence, Tappan revealed his panicked state of mind by using underlines and capital letters to explain his point of view (a style of punctuation this historian has never seen in over a decade of examining the records of the U.S. Public Health Service): "WHAT WILL I DO ABOUT JUAREZ?"[39]

A few days later, Dr. B. J. Lloyd, who served as the medical officer for the U.S. Department of Labor in El Paso, offered a more even-tempered assessment of the local typhus situation at the surgeon general's request. Typhus, he explained calmly, existed in many American cities but was not likely to "become a serious menace to our civilian population." While Dr. Lloyd agreed that erecting a new steam disinfection plant and hiring additional medical manpower were wise measures, he also expressed strong disapproval about the way the public health officers in El Paso were approaching the crisis: "Frankly, the sooner I am relieved from any responsibility for this muddling, the happier I will be."[40] In a subsequent letter to the surgeon general, Lloyd warned that the plan of gasoline bathing every Mexican who crossed the border was likely to cause far more problems than the ones Drs. Tappan and Pierce proposed to solve.[41]

The squabbles over strategy and health control in Texas did little to address the more serious problems being experienced in Mexico itself. In late August 1916, Charles Montague, a former American consular agent and the president of a mining company based in the Mexican province of Sonora, traveled to Chihuahua. Once there, both Villa's revolutionary brigade and the local typhus fever epidemic unnerved him. Montague described one small town where more than fifty typhus deaths occurred each day, resulting in a mass exodus of impoverished Mexican families. Many of these travelers fled in overcrowded and unsanitary railroad cars, and were in poor health, emaciated, and compelled to leave their homes in order "to escape death either by starvation or typhus."

Yet the saddest passage from Montague's typhus diary portrays a fleeing family whose three-month-old baby died of the infection during the long train ride up to El Paso:

> The parents were sent to the cemetery about two miles distant to inter the unfortunate creature. Before the parents returned, the train pulled out, leaving them behind, notwithstanding efforts on the part of the passengers that, when the parents of the dead infant had gone to bury their babe, they left four or five other children on the train, without friends, provisions or money.[42]

If typhus was going to come to Texas, Montague wrote Dr. Tappan, it would be in the bodies of "thousands of peons who are daily coming to the border and crossing to the American side."[43]

During the summer and fall of 1916, unproductive disagreements continued to escalate between the many different federal agencies stationed in the area. It was one thing for public health doctors like Pierce to write letters proposing a twelve-day quarantine for all Mexican immigrants (the incubation period for a budding case of typhus fever), it was quite another to secure the necessary funding to build and staff the detention camps to house them. Some politicians suggested that the U.S. Army troops already in the area undertake this public health mission. Conversely, the United States Army felt it had enough to do with its unofficial war against Mexico and Pancho Villa without patrolling the border against typhus.[44] In turn, the Mexican government was doubly outraged not only by the presence of General John J. Pershing's troops but also by the tacit assumption of their American neighbors that the disease originated exclusively from their country. Tragicomically, the Mexican Board of Health ordered a retaliatory quarantine against all goods and persons arriving from New York City, some 2,500 miles away, where a deadly epidemic of poliomyelitis was raging.[45]

One person who did try to wage a caring and effective campaign against typhus fever in El Paso during 1916 was an earnest physician with the unfortunate name of William C. Kluttz. Each morning the thirty-nine-year-old doctor, who earned his living as a public health physician for the El Paso Board of Health, kissed his wife, Josephine, and his two daughters, Josephine Jr., eight, and Jane, three, goodbye and drove to Chihuahuita. Once there, he inspected its tenements, water wells, and streets, and provided medical care for those residents who required attention.

Born in Salisbury, North Carolina, in 1877, Kluttz received his bachelor's degree at the University of North Carolina in 1896 and his medical degree from one of the nation's premier medical schools, the University of Pennsylvania, in 1899. Afterward, Kluttz remained in Philadelphia for several years, training as an internist and pathologist. But like many young physicians of this era, Kluttz contracted tuberculosis. How he actually got TB is unclear. He may have been infected while treating his patients, during the course of performing an autopsy in the "dead house," or, given the high incidence of tuberculosis in the late nineteenth century, he may simply have contracted it from a friend or acquaintance. Regardless of the source, his aspirations for a prestigious medical career were effectively dashed. And so Dr. Kluttz left the City of Brotherly Love, traveled to the Southwest, and finally settled in El Paso, which was recommended to him by his physician for its healing climate, dry air, and opportunity. Once his tuberculosis went into remission, Kluttz applied for and received a job as a physician in the El Paso Health Department. A few years later he met the woman who became his wife, and soon after the two began to raise a family.[46]

A week before Christmas in 1916, Dr. Kluttz attended the sickbeds of three Mexicans living in Chihuahuita who had recently arrived in El Paso from a war-torn region of Mexico. Kluttz was alerted to this group by another Mexican resident who often served as his translator and scout for the sum of twenty-five cents a day. The three Mexicans appeared quite ill, with spots all over their bodies and high fevers. "Could the newcomers be suffering from *el tabardillo*?" asked Kluttz's assistant. After a brief examination of Maria Pallares, age thirteen, Pablo Pardo, sixteen, and his older brother Ernesto, twenty-six, Dr. Kluttz was certain that they did indeed have typhus fever.

The public health physician placed the three Mexicans under quarantine, arranged to bring rations of food and water, and volunteered to make daily visits. Dr. Kluttz, of course, had a great deal of experience in caring for typhus patients, and was usually careful to disinfect and wash himself after each visit. But something must have gone amiss with his sterile technique after one of these house calls. On the way back to his office on the afternoon of December 19 or 20, Dr. Kluttz reported feeling a sharp, stinging sensation in the groin area. Might it have been a louse bite? By the evening of the twenty-second, it seemed almost certain that he had encountered a rickettsial-filled louse, because upon returning home that evening, he declined his favorite dinner, baked pork chops and fried potatoes, and instead took to his bed feeling feverish and ill.

El Paso's finest physicians came out day and night to attend to their comrade. But the typhus he encountered was of a particularly virulent variety and Kluttz was dead by January 4, 1917. He was lauded in the El Paso newspapers as a martyr to science, and his death became a unifying call to arms to do something once and for all against typhus and its presumed importer, Mexican immigrants. No one expressed this charge better than the mayor of El Paso, Tom Lea, as he presided over Dr. Kluttz's funeral. Calling Dr. Kluttz's death a "needless sacrifice," Mayor Lea castigated the bureaucrats in Washington, D.C., for refusing to enact "a strong, federally controlled quarantine here that would effectively stop the entrance into this country of disease-bearing persons from south of the Rio Grande." Such public health efforts might have cost the government "a little money" or wounded "the sensitive feelings of our neighbors," Lea eulogized, but Dr. Kluttz's life, not to mention the welfare of all of El Paso's citizenry, might have been protected had they only listened to his sensible medical advice.[47]

The news of Dr. Kluttz's death quickly made its way to Washington, D.C., where Surgeon General Rupert Blue, after months of mulling the situation over, finally ordered Drs. Pierce and Tappan to coordinate medical inspection efforts along the entire Texas border, with stations at El Paso, Eagle Pass, Laredo, Rio Grande City, and Brownsville. Only Eagle Pass and Laredo had operable steam disinfection plants in early 1917. Dissatisfied by the cordon sanitaire of medical inspections and selective steam disinfections, Pierce and Tappan ruled that *every* Mexican passing the border be subjected to a mandatory delousing bath in a mixture of gasoline, kerosene, and vinegar. The doctors even had special certificates printed up by Alamo Printing Company which the bathed Mexicans were required to carry with them at all times in the event they were questioned.[48] On January 23, 1917, the same week President Wilson ordered Pershing to withdraw his troops from Mexico, Pierce sent a circular, approved by the surgeon general, to all USPHS officers stationed along the Texas-Mexico border, as well as those in Naco, Nogales, Douglas, and Tucson, Arizona. It decreed the strict closure of the border to Mexican traffic every night and the mandatory bathing and medical inspection of all Mexicans each day to prevent the entry of typhus, effective January 27 at 7 p.m.[49] All of these abrupt changes in policy proved to be almost as explosive as the bathing mixture itself.

A t seven o'clock in the morning on January 28, a Juárez–El Paso streetcar carrying a group of Mexican women was stopped in the middle of the Santa Fe Bridge, the point where Mexico ended and the United States began. The USPHS assistant surgeon, Dr. C. C. Pierce, boarded the streetcar and ordered the women to leave the car quietly and enter the disinfecting building just off the side of the bridge. As Pierce later remarked to a reporter for the *El Paso Morning Times:* "the greater part of them refused to go along." One Mexican observer had a reasonable explanation for the women's lack of cooperation: "their indignation increased once they were ordered off the street cars, after having paid their fares and could not have their nickels refunded."[50]

Soon after Pierce explained the details of the quarantine order, the women complained that they would suffer financial consequences from reporting late to their daily jobs or prospective employers. But as the public health physician ordered them to line up single file for the mandatory gasoline-kerosene-vinegar baths, their anger and fear grew with each passing moment. All protests need a leader, someone to agitate a group of disgruntled individuals into a mob with force. That morning the task fell to a seventeen-year-old named Carmela "Carmelita" Torres, who came to be referred to in both the local and national press covering the event as "the Auburn-haired Amazon."[51]

Carmelita was a spirited young woman who earned her living washing the clothes, cleaning the house, and feeding and minding the children of a wealthy businessman in El Paso. She was paid approximately five dollars a week for her labor, but back in Juárez this was enough to help significantly in feeding her family and paying the rent. She had been working as a domestic servant since she was twelve. There were, of course, many Carmelitas working in the homes of well-to-do El Pasoans. Ironically, the same people who grumbled the loudest about the threat of Mexican-imported typhus and other diseases thought little of these dangers when meals needed to be cooked, laundry washed, or children readied for bed, a dissonant reality of American attitudes toward foreign labor that continues up to the present.[52]

A mob of angry people, as Charles Dickens once observed in the climactic scene of *Oliver Twist,* is a distinct living entity of its own. Like an epidemic, no one can predict how it will take shape or proceed. One can only fully comprehend its course after the dust settles. On the morning of January 28, the Mexican women's response to the quarantine essentially started with Carmelita's crude and witty jeers. Caught up in the excitement of the moment, she refused to stop with a few quips. As one observer noted, Torres "kept up a continuous volley of language aimed at the immigration and health officers, civilians and sentries and any other visible Americans."[53]

But beyond mere catcalls, many other inciting factors helped to shape the tumultuous events that transpired. Anti-American sentiments over the recent occupation of Mexico by the U.S. Army, reactions to being labeled "diseased," and the strict quarantine with its gasoline baths (which the Juárez residents knew led to the deaths of twenty-six prisoners only nine months earlier) all contributed to the Mexicans' anger. So, too, did the rumors that American officials would be photographing the women—their wives, sisters, and mothers—as they disrobed for the delousing baths. Certainly, all of these resentments transformed the event from a shouting match begun by Carmelita and her co-workers into something far more dangerous. Soon, one of the workers threw some stones at the guards. Glass bottles began to fly, and it was not long before a full-scale riot ensued.

The initial crowd of two hundred protesters quickly swelled to more than a thousand. The enraged mob was now predominantly male, fueled by alcohol, and shouted its support for Pancho Villa. Some of the women and men, who were waiting on the Juárez side of the closed bridge, decided they would cross the border regardless of the quarantine order. They jumped down onto the sandy banks of the Rio Grande, only to be captured and beaten by guards. Others overturned the streetcars that ran between Juárez and El Paso, and pulled out the conductors and streetcar operators, beating some senseless.[54]

Fortunately, no one was killed, but many people on both sides of the melee were seriously injured. By mid-afternoon, the El Paso and Juárez jails were filled to capacity, and armed guards on both sides of the border threatened to retaliate if provoked. The mayor of Juárez, Melchor Herrera, called these policies an "unjust measure, caused undoubtedly by the malevolence of our enemies, who never lose an opportunity to publicly proclaim the most stupendous notices in regard to the condition of our public health." Nevertheless, Mayor Herrera urged his fellow citizens to calm down, avoid violence, and trust their "popular representatives" to find a suitable compromise.[55]

Despite this mayoral advice, the people of Juárez had one more riot in them, and the following morning, January 29, hundreds of Mexican laborers approached the barricaded entrance of the Santa Fe International Bridge armed with milk bottles, stones, and anything else they could throw. But the element of surprise was gone and hundreds of U.S. soldiers were prepared to meet them on the other side with orders to use their rifles if the protest got out of control. It did not, and by afternoon the Mexicans who needed to cross acquiesced and consented to the baths. As one Juárez resident recalled decades later, the decision was not a complicated one: "It was a requirement for anyone who wanted to work."[56]

The haggling over the quarantine continued in the months that followed the riot. Juárez officials and Mexican consulate officers thought it was too harsh and, of course, the USPHS physicians stationed in El Paso thought it was not strict enough. As Dr. Pierce insisted in a letter to the surgeon general that February, typhus germs entered the United States exclusively in the bodies of illegal aliens who "crossed the bridge at Juárez–El Paso at night, on the cars or walking, claiming to be 'locals,' and have thus evaded disinfection and have spread the disease in El Paso and other places."[57]

Eventually, a compromise of sorts was reached: the quarantine against Mexican immigrants continued, but dayworkers were required to be bathed, steamed, and disinfected once a week rather than daily, provided they had a valid "disinfection certificate" signed by a USPHS officer. Carmelita and her colleagues decided it was easier to cooperate than to riot.

The magnitude of medical inspections performed during this period was staggering. Between January 13 and June 9, 1917, a skeleton crew of physicians conducted 871,639 medical examinations of immigrants and dayworkers. From this throng, 402 were excluded because of some type of illness, 7 were denied entry for refusing disinfection, and 8 were held for observation. Interestingly, 31 cases of typhus fever were reported in the entire United States during this six-month period and only 3 of them were discovered in El Paso.[58]

Repeated requests were made throughout 1917 to relax the typhus vigil—especially since no cases of infection were discovered after May of that year—but to no avail, and the quarantine against the incursion of typhus from Mexico remained in effect until the 1930s. Disinfection plants were eventually built at all of the other Texas-Mexico quarantine stations as well as in New Mexico and Arizona.[59]

In fact, there is excellent documentation that by 1920 what was once the most lax immigrant inspection process in the United States became one of the tightest.[60] About 90 percent of the arrivals to the border during this period were classified as impoverished refugees, and were subjected to mandatory full medical examinations, smallpox vaccinations, and delousing steam baths.[61] Yet once settled, the health and living conditions immigrants experienced in ghettos like El Paso's Chihuahuita or New York's Lower East Side remained every bit as dangerous as they were in the years leading up to these regulatory changes.

Today, typhus may not be the major health threat that it once was, but it still manages to travel great distances, especially when accompanied by war and impoverished living conditions. Nor has it lost its ability to inspire devastating assaults on the health of those who come in its path. In the immediate years before, during, and after World War I, typhus fever managed to infect 20 to 30 million people and killed several million including our semi-reliable correspondent John Reed, who died of it in Moscow in 1920.[62] During World War II the germ killed at least 3 million more people.[63] Most recently, typhus appeared in the aftermath of the U.S.-Iraq war in 1990, where it was most ruthless in attacking Iraqi children under the age of ten; in Bosnia, where notorious efforts at "ethnic cleansing" unfolded during the late 1990s; and currently in South America and Africa, particularly the nations of Ethiopia, Burundi, and Rwanda, where it kills between 30,000 and 60,000 people a year.

Nevertheless, the American approach to containing typhus in the years before World War I does provide a cautionary tale. To be sure, the transformation of the vague Mexican-U.S. border from an imaginary line drawn in the desert to a patrolled boundary emerged out of concerns over national sovereignty, economics, and racial differences. But the threat of typhus, the fear that "Mexican disease" might enter the United States, helped hold it together.

Almost a decade after the typhus riot, Dr. Tappan proudly documented the "successful" 2,000-mile quarantine he erected along the Mexican border in the *Journal of the American Medical Association* and reminded his medical colleagues: "Conditions differ from those on the Canadian border. We have here to contend with an alien race; one with a different language, different customs, different moral standards, and different diseases."[64] The relatively low incidence of typhus or any other epidemic disease imported into the United States from Mexico during this period can be interpreted two ways: either the harsh inspection and disinfection methods were effective, or the threat was not nearly as large as it was thought to be. Undoubtedly, the truth lies somewhere in between.[65]

With the brilliant clarity of hindsight, it is difficult to deny that a huge price was paid for public health measures considered punitive by the immigrants subjected to them. The "jail holocaust" and the subsequent quarantine at El Paso incited Mexicans like Carmelita Torres and her fellow workers to express their resistance in a violent manner. As time went on and the Mexicans appeared to be complying with the quarantine regimen, American officials assumed they had beaten them into compliance. The majority did follow the disinfection and inspection procedures, but we know that there were many others who crossed into the United States at undesignated and illegal points of entry to evade scrutiny. This trend was noted as early as 1921 and ultimately led to the creation of the United States Border Patrol.[66]

Perhaps the most troubling, if unintended, consequence of the efforts to tighten the U.S.-Mexican border and examine those legally crossing it was the subsequent rise of illegal immigrants, some of whom harbored infections or feared medical examinations of any kind. Today, in an era where there are, at least, 250,000 undocumented immigrants entering the United States each year, the threat of imported infection is far more than a theoretical concern. Matters become more serious when considering the deleterious conditions these illegal immigrants often endure while emigrating to and settling in the United States, not to mention the paucity of health care available to them.

Yet, instead of creating the means to promote health on both sides of the Rio Grande, we more often opt for the false sense of security afforded by the construction of walls and immigrant checkpoints along a 2,000-mile-long porous boundary. As our nation invests billions of dollars in surveillance devices and barbed wire, hundreds of thousands of Mexicans and others living on either side of the border live in an environment one reporter for the *New York Times* recently characterized as "a hotbed of contagion."[67] The history of contagious diseases teaches us little if it does not remind us that when we employ mechanisms that deny or frighten away those most in need of medical attention, we create a host of new problems rather than solving the old ones. Indeed, we ignore the basic premise of medical practice that Hippocrates introduced more than 2,500 years ago in a treatise entitled *Epidemics:* "As to diseases, make a habit of two things—to help, or at least, to do no harm."[68]

# FIVE

# No One's Idea of a Tropical Paradise: Haitian Immigrants and AIDS

Often it would start in Port-au-Prince, with drinks at the Palace Hotel or Chez Denis where locals mixed easily with tourists and the rum was deep. An early evening drive would take you past the national palace and the shuttered pastel shops, toward the dilapidated wharf area, along the gutted coastal roads into the poor bidons, or slums, with names such as Cité Simone and Carrefour, the red-light district. . . . Or if one pleased, there was . . . Petionville, where the wealthy white and mulatto minority lived in a fairy-tale existence of restaurants, gambling casinos, and European nightclubs. Behind the wrought-iron gates of private villas, huge parties would take place, the crowds, wild and international. Men from Paris and Africa danced with the local set, old with young, rich with poor, black with white, with mulatto and every shade in between. Anyone might show up: transvestites, bisexuals, voyeurs, prostitutes, boudon (voodoo) priests and even the Tonton Macoutes, the brutal goons of "Papa Doc" Duvalier, out for a good time.

—ANNE-CHRISTINE D'ADESKY[1]

L ate one night in 1992, under a bright full moon, Tomás left Haiti with twenty-nine others fleeing their native land. He first met his fellow travelers only an hour before they shoved off the beach. Their transportation was a boat so patched and flimsy that its safety for a mere fishing trip on a calm lake was questionable, let alone for a 120-mile ocean voyage. But Tomás had little choice. After angering the local authorities in Port-au-Prince by organizing a series of demonstrations in support of the democratically elected, and later militarily deposed, president Jean-Bertrand Aristide, he was forced underground to escape a brutal death. Soon after, he began to raise the money he needed to secure a place on one of the rickety boats that left nightly on the dangerous trip to the United States. Consequently, the seaworthiness of the boat he jumped into was not an issue burning in his mind. In fact, the only thing he could focus upon, besides the annoyingly loud thumping of his heart, was an urgent warning he heard constantly in his head: Run for your life! Escape! Get out of Haiti!

The voyage began badly and ended worse. Tossed about on the rough Atlantic water, Tomás and several others soon became seasick. Some of the passengers began to pray loudly for safety or, at least, a gentle death. The array of rosaries, battered Bibles, and voodoo relics that instantly appeared was the stuff that anthropology graduate students might spend years dissecting for their doctoral theses. Although most Haitians were aware that the waters were routinely patrolled by U.S. Coast Guard ships to prevent their flight, Tomás held onto the hope that his fate

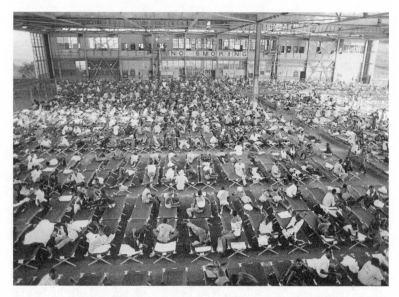

*Haitian refugees are lined up in cots in the McCalla hangar at Guantánamo Bay Naval Base in Cuba, December 5, 1999.*

would be different; that he would elude the radar, telescopes, and search technology of the American patrol boats and manage to reach safety and freedom. And like the tens of thousands of other Haitians who fled during the late 1980s and early 1990s, he was wrong.

Some sixty miles from where they pushed off the Haitian beach, the blinding searchlights of a Coast Guard cutter aimed directly at the tiny vessel carrying Tomás and his countrymen. The thirty refugees were brought aboard the cutter, given blankets and coffee, and escorted to a section of the ship below the main deck. Tomás was astounded to find about a hundred other Haitians on board who had already been intercepted that night. The Coast Guard crew continued its mission and gathered up five more boats, carrying approximately 150 Haitians, before turning their ship's bow to the southern tip of Cuba—the U.S. naval base at Guantánamo Bay, which was the site of a giant Haitian refugee camp.

When the cutter docked off the bay and naval personnel escorted Tomás and his fellow travelers ashore the following morning, they were confused and exhausted. The crowds of Haitians on the island were initially reassuring, but soon enough the newcomers realized that the camp was a virtual sea of Haitians, tents, barbed wire, and armed guards. Their dreams of escape faded quickly as they were processed and medically examined, including testing for evidence of infection with the human immunodeficiency virus (HIV).

The American story of human migration and AIDS actually begins six years earlier in 1986. That year, Senator Jesse Helms (R–North Carolina), a noted opponent of gay rights and AIDS programs, introduced an amendment to a bill that specifically banned HIV-positive immigrants or foreign visitors from entering the United States. President George H. W. Bush's secretary of health, Louis Sullivan, himself a widely respected physician, disagreed with this policy, arguing that only immigrants with tuberculosis should be barred because, unlike AIDS or other sexually transmitted diseases, tuberculosis was truly "a communicable disease of public health significance." Dr. Sullivan's medical opinion was ignored, however, and the federal regulation initiated by Helms stayed in effect until 1991. That year the policy was changed only slightly: HIV-positive tourists or "travelers" could enter the United States, but immigrants wishing to settle permanently were banned. *All* immigrants seeking a temporary visa were required to report to the United States Embassy in their nation of origin and be tested for HIV; those seeking asylum at an American port or border were allowed to live in the United States for a year while their case was adjudicated, but they, too, were required to submit to an HIV test. The overall message was clear: those who could afford to travel as tourists, regardless of HIV status, were begrudgingly welcome. Those impoverished and potentially ill immigrants "likely to become a public charge" were not.[2]

By early 1992, survival rather than AIDS was the chief concern for Haitians attempting to escape to the United States. On his first day at Guantánamo, Tomás rolled up his sleeve and a naval medical corpsman inserted a sharp syringe into one of the spongy veins jutting out of his forearm to extract enough blood for the mandatory HIV test. But instead of thinking about the specter of incurable disease, Tomás's immediate thoughts focused on the quick removal of the needle.

Days went by before Tomás was called back to the doctor's office for his test results. Escorted by two guards whose hands were carefully poised on their automatic rifles, Tomás nervously sat on the other side of what he later recalled to be an enormous metallic desk. The doctor's body movements and vocal pattern seemed to Tomás to be occurring in slow motion. So distorted was the physician's voice, as Tomás heard it, that he initially refused to believe the diagnostic pronouncement being delivered. "It seems that there is a slight problem with your blood," the doctor drawled. "Our laboratory tests tell us that you have been infected with AIDS."

Tomás remained on Guantánamo for almost two years before he was finally admitted into the United States. For most of that time he adamantly denied being HIV-positive. This was a claim quite common among the approximately 255 Haitians detained in a place that could be described only as an HIV/AIDS prison camp. Tomás had to search his memory for the date he left his tiny village or the night he left Haiti entirely, but for the remaining days of his life, he could always summon up the exact day and time when he was first told about the "slight problem" with his blood test.

N ot terribly long ago, every schoolchild used to recite the doggerel verse "In 1492, Columbus sailed the ocean blue." And while such poetic attempts are no longer in vogue, let alone the so-called discoverers who inspired them, it is worth noting that in 1492 Christopher Columbus did land on the northern coast of an island he named Hispaniola. For those whose memories of first-grade geography may be somewhat dim, the western one-third of this island constitutes Haiti and the remainder is the Dominican Republic.

When Admiral Columbus triumphantly visited the court of Queen Isabella and King Ferdinand in April 1493, he was asked to describe what Hispaniola looked like. Columbus is said to have reached for a piece of paper from the queen's writing desk, wadded it up into a ball, and replied: "It looks like that." Whether an actual historical event or apocryphal tale, the Columbus anecdote does reflect the oft-repeated Haitian expression that is used to describe both the rugged landscape and the difficult life of Haiti: "it looks like mountains and more mountains."[3]

The ratio of human beings to acreage of arable land in Haiti is one of the highest on the planet. The abrupt mountainsides are particularly inhospitable to nurturing crops of any kind. Despite ambitious attempts to overcultivate what little land does welcome vegetation, the island has its own perverse methods of fighting back. Each year more of Haiti's precious topsoil slides into the sea, leaving a somewhat lunar landscape behind. In concert with this terrestrial movement off the island, many Haitians emigrate to other nations.[4]

The majority of Haitians remain in the underdeveloped countryside of the island working tiny plots of land, often smaller than an acre or two, with little more farming technology than that employed by their ancestors: their muscular backs and a machete. The official language is Creole-French, and while Haiti's official religion is Catholicism, many practice voodoo. Family structure is looser knit than elsewhere in the Western Hemisphere. In Haiti, men often live in common-law marriages with women, several if they have the means. Foreigners are looked at with great suspicion, and to many peasants, this includes city dwellers, who are often better educated, wealthier, and may be mulatto in racial composition.[5]

When contemplating Haiti's vital statistics, it is difficult not to become depressed. Just as the paucity of fertile land makes food production arduous, the country's oppressive poverty, low levels of education, and periodic violent sprees of political and social disruption are the perfect soil for myriad public health problems. The average per capita income during the late 1980s and early 1990s was less than $350 per year. The unemployment rate was about 80 percent. Looking at the two most sensitive indicators of a nation's health and well-being, one would not be surprised to learn that Haiti has the highest infant mortality rate and the second lowest life-expectancy rate in the Western Hemisphere. Few official reports state the Haitian health situation more bleakly than those produced annually by UNICEF: in 1985, for example, a child died every five minutes, and problems such as malnutrition and infectious diseases long since conquered in other parts of the Western world were daily visitors to the Haitian people.[6] Finally, there is another major factor to be considered that is both obvious and rarely discussed: the color of its people. Haiti is primarily a nation of people of African descent, many of whom were originally brought there because of the slave trade, and it is essential to consider its public health problems and international relations through the murky prism of race.[7]

Haiti's historical trajectory from the days of Columbus to the present has been strikingly tempestuous. It is a land, in the words of one historian, "which has been the theater of such horrible scenes and frightful dramas, whose soil has drunk more blood than sweat." After being established as a principal way station in the slave trade, Haiti became an important part of Napoleon's empire, generating more wealth for France from the cultivation of coffee beans than all of its other colonies combined. Violent revolt, which has come to characterize this troubled spot in the Caribbean, began in the eighteenth century. Led by a former slave named Toussaint L'Ouverture, who was inspired by the principles of freedom and the "rights of man" espoused during the French Revolution, Haiti became Latin America's first self-declared independent nation in 1804 and, outside of Africa, the first to be led by blacks. This racial demographic made Haiti an especially sore spot among slaveholders in the United States and Europe, and many large nations refused to recognize the new republic long after its official independence.[8]

In the decades that followed, Haiti became only more violent and troubled. Its timeline is marred by slavery, colonization, war, coups d'état, mass murder, and generalized chaos, with only the names of those in leadership and the sources of outside interference changing. For purposes of our exploration of the relationship of the AIDS epidemic to Haitian society, however, one needs to examine the regime of François "Papa Doc" Duvalier. Duvalier became president of Haiti in 1957 and stayed in that position until his death in 1971, when his then nineteen-year-old son, Jean-Claude "Baby Doc" Duvalier, succeeded him.[9]

If only two words were chosen to describe the Duvaliers' reign, "tyranny" and "corruption" would immediately come to mind. Most infamous was Papa Doc's institution of the Tonton Macoutes, a cadre of rural headsmen, or *chefs de section,* who constituted a militia that took on the traits of a religious sect, political party, quasi-Gestapo, and terrorist cell. The Tonton Macoutes not only worked on behalf of President Duvalier but also to enrich themselves at the expense of Haiti's peasant population. A 1964 issue of *The New Republic* described the very model of a modern Tonton Macoute as "a Duvalier activist. In 99 cases out of 100 he is black. The civilian Tonton Macoute can be recognized by his sharp clothes, dark glasses, pearl-gray homburg, and the bulge of a pistol on his hip. . . . This man is an informer, neighborhood boss, extortioner, bully, and political pillar of the regime."[10]

Over the years, their uniforms changed somewhat, but the power of the Duvaliers and their henchmen became only more absolute. The Tonton Macoutes took what they wanted, be it food, goods, services, money, personal possessions, and, if the urge struck them, sexual favors. Refusals were construed as a hostile act to the Duvalier government, and these "uncooperative citizens" were at a minimum beaten and jailed or, all too often, killed in plain sight of others. With the growing corruption under Papa Doc, Haiti sank lower and lower into poverty and despair. The national ethos of despotism only intensified in 1971 with his son's ascension to the presidency. Baby Doc Duvalier, as one reporter wrote, looked at Haiti as a private possession for the advancement of his personal pleasure and insatiable hedonism. He was always "ready to sell the country to the highest bidder."[11] The Haitians had an expression for his dictatorship named after a popular frozen snack, *peze-suce,* or "squeeze and suck."[12] When Jean-Claude Duvalier and his wife were driven into exile in 1986, the legacy they left behind was one of utter social turmoil, poverty, agony, and disease.

T wo major developments accompanied the last few decades of Duvalierism. The first was increased migration from the impoverished villages into the cities or off the island entirely. The second was a burgeoning tourism industry that came to an abrupt halt by 1982 with the initial recognition of AIDS.

During the 1960s, Haitian officials aggressively promoted the island as a tourist destination. For example, in a welcoming speech to Nelson Rockefeller, who was serving as President Richard M. Nixon's Latin American envoy in 1969, Papa Doc Duvalier disingenuously boasted: "Haiti could be a great kind of relaxation for the American middle class—it is close, beautiful, and politically stable." By the beginning of the 1970s, Port-au-Prince had become a popular day-docking station for several American and European cruise ship lines. In fact, during these years tourism was well on its way to surpassing coffee and the country's many offshore assembly plants as Haiti's chief source of income. Before 1960, fewer than 30,000 tourists ventured annually to Haiti. By 1979, more than 150,000 came to Haiti for vacations, not counting the day visitors from cruise lines. The following year, 1980, the numbers increased twofold with the opening of a lavish Club Méditerranée resort.[13] But with tourism came a spirit of good times, and the combination of wealthy visitors and impoverished islanders led to a burgeoning prostitution industry.

Haiti was an especially popular vacation spot for members of the gay community—both American and European. Just before the initial outbreak of AIDS, the 1981 *Spartacus International Gay Guide* extolled Haiti's freewheeling party scene, the Haitians' "easy-going attitude towards sex in general," and the abundance of "well-endowed" men "with a great ability to satisfy whatever it is you are looking for." Ranking Haiti as one of the world's "top ten" gay vacation destinations, the guide concluded: "If you are turned on by beautiful black guys, and you can adjust to Haiti's extreme poverty and lack of creature comforts, you may indeed find Haiti a paradise."[14]

In the more than twenty years since the first baffling cases of what we call the acquired immune deficiency syndrome (AIDS) captured the attention of the medical community and lay public alike, there has been much discussion in countless books and articles about where and how AIDS originated.[15] This query holds a fascination that is far out of proportion to other critical issues surrounding the epidemic's control and the treatment of those infected with HIV.

Such ultimately aimless searches for the origins of a specific contagious disease hardly began with AIDS. Only four centuries earlier, the sexually transmitted disease syphilis was widely believed to be among the many things Christopher Columbus brought back with him from Hispaniola to Spain. By the mid-sixteenth century, medical professors across Europe espoused elegant theories on the American origins of syphilis. In 1564 the esteemed Italian physician Gabrielo Fallopio, who identified the tubes that lead from the ovaries to the uterus and bear his name, wrote a thesis explaining that Columbus may have discovered a new continent filled with "untold islands, uncouth slaves, and treasures of gold and silver, but that the precious metals concealed a thorn . . . the soldiers who returned to Europe were laden more with sickness than with gold, and they passed the curse onto others who took up military service with the Italian expeditions at the time of the siege of Naples."[16] During this period syphilis was alternatively referred to as the "Spanish disease," the "Italian evil," or the "French pox," depending largely upon those charged with labeling it and those being labeled.

In the late seventeenth century, the eminent British physician Sir Thomas Sydenham, still reverentially referred to as the "English Hippocrates," reported that Europe's syphilis "problem" was chiefly a result of the transport of black slaves from Africa to America, and that, in turn, the disease was brought to the Old World by the slave traders. In reality, Sydenham was a far better observer of his patients' illnesses than he was an interpreter of history. The initial transport of slaves from Africa to America took place between 1503 and 1508. The first recorded outbreak of syphilis in Europe was 1495.[17] But while the origin of syphilis remains disputed to this very day, it is an excellent lesson of how the shroud of blame can be confusing, misleading, and entirely beside the point of protecting the public health.

During the first decade of the AIDS epidemic, many theories were developed linking its origin to gay sexual practices, specific drugs of abuse, and, with respect to Haiti, voodoo blood rituals. But in the case of Haiti, if AIDS did not originate on the island, it did not randomly appear there either. Specific social, cultural, economic, and medical circumstances were necessary in order for the epidemic to reach its shores.

The French historian Mirko Grmek coined the term "pathocenosis" to describe the development and frequency of disease affecting a particular population at a specific point in history. Pathocenosis typically remains in equilibrium in "a relatively closed and ecologically stable population." These equilibrium states can be disrupted easily by major demographic upheavals such as the shift from active to sedentary lifestyles among humans during the Neolithic period, the migration of people from Asia to the West during the Middle Ages, the European discovery of America during the Renaissance, and the creation of the global village that characterizes our era. Not surprisingly, one of the most glaring consequences of these historic social ruptures has been the outbreak of deadly epidemics.[18] The virus that causes AIDS had likely been around for decades or longer before physicians recognized its manifestations during the early 1980s. But something in its genetic structure probably mutated or changed drastically to transmogrify the microbe that once resided quietly in several species of primates to the deadly agent we encounter today. In concert with these mutations or changes in pathogenicity, however, were a number of disrupting social shifts that helped AIDS travel more widely, including the sexual revolution of the 1960s and 1970s. These decades saw a huge increase in sexual promiscuity, anonymous sexual contacts, freedom from worries over pregnancy with the advent of oral contraception, and the increased incidence of sexually transmitted diseases among both the gay and heterosexual communities. It was also an era that witnessed a boom in international travel, making an infection of HIV in, say, Paris, easily transferable to New York or San Francisco. The point here is not to make a moral judgment on sexual mores among a particular adult community. Instead, it is merely to demonstrate that changes in behavior, be they sexual, social, or cultural, can contribute to a pathocenotic wave.[19]

As opposed to a place of origin, Haiti was, most likely, a stopover point in the progress of the AIDS pandemic. Given today's knowledge of where and when the earliest cases of AIDS were recognized, epidemiologists have hypothesized that this tour probably began somewhere in

Central Africa and then extended from that continent to Europe and the United States. The virus subsequently traveled into Haiti in the bodies of wayfarers or Haitians who had made visits to Africa, the United States, or Europe. Tomás, the Haitian refugee interned on Guantánamo, presents an excellent example of the complicated path of HIV during these years.[20]

Like most Haitian men, Tomás categorically denied being homosexual.[21] However, he did admit to a career as a male prostitute for the pleasure-hungry tourist trade during the late 1970s. He initially insisted that his clients were primarily women, and men only if the money was tight. But on further questioning, Tomás acknowledged that almost all of his customers were men, chiefly from Europe but also New York, San Francisco, Los Angeles, and other large American cities.

When he left his village for Port-au-Prince in late 1977, Tomás was seventeen years old. Initially, he simply hoped to make enough money to return to his hometown and set up a small grocery store or, better yet, have enough to emigrate to the United States, where he had family in Brooklyn, New York. But it did not take long for Tomás to appreciate that his good looks, outgoing and pleasant personality, and charm were his most valuable assets. The party scene during these years in places like Port-au-Prince, Cap Haitien on the north coast, and Jacmel in the south was, to say the least, incredible. Food, wine, drugs, and sex flowed as freely as the ocean breeze. In Port-au-Prince, Tomás met several other ambitious young men who had migrated from mountain villages to the city. These friends, many of whom were already engaged in the gay sex trade, advised him that such work was both easy and lucrative. All he had to do was to close his eyes and allow the sexual events to transpire. The johns even provided plentiful supplies of rum, marijuana, and cocaine, if Tomás needed to be inebriated to make these episodes more tolerable.

Quickly establishing himself as a beach boy, Tomás started his day in the late afternoon, after his potential customers had a chance to finish lunch and begin their odyssey into drunkenness. Dressed in a tank top and swimming shorts that displayed his tall muscular body at its best, Tomás soon became a popular figure. Sometimes on slow days, Tomás would have to approach clients for sexual encounters of the commercial kind, but more often than not they approached him. The propositions were rarely verbally articulated. A long glance over the top of his sunglasses, a volley of smiles and winks, and a signal for the customer to follow him to a clandestine spot, or a hotel room that was rented by the hour, constituted the language of these transactions. But there were two other exchanges that would have great import to Tomás. The first, of course, was immediate: money for a sexual favor; the second one he would not have to grapple with until a decade later: the exchange of body fluids—some of which must have carried the HIV virus into his body.

There were too many men for Tomás actually to count, let alone identify as the precise source of his infection. Whether it was someone he met at the beach or at the wild nightly parties he attended while under the influence of drugs and alcohol, the two living entities, HIV and Tomás, met. More than fourteen years later, the question of who introduced him to the human immunodeficiency virus was something Tomás thought about almost every day.

Not all Haitians who contracted HIV did so, however, by gay sex. Some women were infected by promiscuous husbands or may have engaged in the sex trade themselves. Others may have been infected because of tainted blood transfusions. In any case, most epidemiologists have concluded that it is extremely unlikely (if not outright impossible) that HIV developed de novo in Haiti any more than syphilis five centuries earlier.

On October 19, 1897, the era's favorite guide to all things medical, Dr. William Osler, was slated to present a lecture in the auditorium of the New York Academy of Medicine. That evening he attracted a standing-room crowd with a talk entitled "Internal Medicine as a Vocation." Osler, a charismatic speaker who was always properly dressed in a frock coat and sported a perfectly groomed handlebar mustache, ambled up to the podium, sipped from a glass of water, and began his address. Before long, he offered his medical colleagues some wise advice: "Know syphilis in all its manifestations and relations and all other things clinical will be added unto you."[22]

Today, of course, we know a great deal more about syphilis than the doctors listening to Osler's lecture that fall evening. But it was not until 1905 that two German physicians named Fritz Schaudinn and Erich Hoffmann identified a furtive bacterium that looks a bit like a corkscrew, *Treponema pallidum,* as the cause of syphilis. So when Osler delivered his famous lecture, American physicians were as puzzled about the exact cause of syphilis as their successors would be almost a century later when the first cases of AIDS were reported.

To be sure, these nineteenth-century physicians understood that syphilis was primarily sexually transmitted, although sensibilities of the era often prevented them from exclaiming this fact too loudly. It was also known to have several stages, three to be exact. The initial stage of infection is typically marked by a painless sore, or chancre, on the genitals, which serves as a reliable marker of where the *Treponema pallidum* first penetrated the body. The sore mysteriously disappears a few weeks later, convincing many infected people that their night of passion was worth the risk after all.

Some six to eight weeks later, a person infected with syphilis enters into the disease's secondary stage, which tends to mimic the symptoms of a bad cold: achiness, malaise, low-grade fevers, a sore throat, and enlarged lymph nodes. But something novel is added to the pathological mix: a curious rash advances over one's ribs and torso before spreading to the rest of the body (but usually sparing the face), accompanied by a crop of itchy, scaly red bumps that develop on the palms of the hands and soles of the feet. This phase soon disappears, although about 25 percent of the microbe's prey develop relapsing skin rashes throughout their lives. And with each resolution, the crafty organism lulls its victim into complacency, falsely assuring that all is fine and that the strange symptoms were minor and self-limiting. For those of us concerned with epidemics, the real problem arises from the fact that people with primary or secondary syphilis are quite contagious to others and can easily spread the disease with the simple act of sexual intercourse.

Yet it is the third phase of syphilis that is the most baffling. If left untreated, the corkscrew-shaped germs burrow their way into critical organs of the body, slowly, bit by bit, destroying them over a course of decades. They leave behind a trail of lesions called gummas, soft, gumlike patches of dead, wasted tissue that appear in the aorta, making this Mississippi of the arterial system likely to dissect and burst; in the brain, causing havoc in the way its victims think, speak, walk, and move; or in the lungs, skin, liver, and bones, to name but a few favorite targets. Hence, William Osler's advice to his fellow physicians that by studying syphilis in all of its manifestations, they would learn a great deal about the human body.

If Dr. Osler were teaching medicine in the twenty-first century, he could just as easily urge his students, "Know HIV/AIDS in all its manifestations and relations and all other things clinical will be added unto you." A virus that has a devastating impact on almost every cell, tissue, and organ it meets as it races through the body, HIV is relentless in its attack and remarkably versatile in its presentation. Especially in the years before the advent of effective anti-retroviral medications, some descended rapidly into horrible illness, while others seemed to remain completely healthy for years. Over the past decade I have treated hundreds of patients with HIV/AIDS, and no two cases have been exactly alike.

Today, so much is known about the biology, pathology, and treatment of AIDS that it seems hard to believe what a frightening mystery it was when it first came to wide attention during the early 1980s. But while most American physicians eschewed the epidemic and its initial victims, many others were inspired to search for the cause and cure of a new disease.[23] As Dr. Paul Volberding, the chief of oncology at the University of California at San Francisco, recalled, joining the early battle against AIDS was like signing up to be a crew member of Columbus's voyage to the New World. It was a scientific journey mixed with equal parts discovery, exhilaration, and fear: "You go through medicine and you expect that everything has been pretty much described and that you'll make progress, and you'll make discoveries, but they're going to be incremental advances in areas that are pretty well outlined. But here there was no history. We were it."[24]

The microbe that causes AIDS, the human immunodeficiency virus (HIV), is not a hearty organism. If you were to leave a droplet of infected body fluid on a tabletop or a toilet seat, the virus would be dead in the time it took for the fluid it was sitting in to dry. Parenthetically, the public toilet seat with its U-shaped configuration was specifically designed in the early twentieth century as a misguided means of preventing the possible spread of sexually transmitted diseases like gonorrhea and syphilis via sitting in the wrong place. Despite years of clinical experience and scientific knowledge of just how difficult it is actually to contract diseases like gonorrhea or syphilis, let alone AIDS, from a toilet seat, the U-shaped lid remains a staple of the American public restroom.[25]

HIV is typically transmitted by sexual activity, but not all activities are equal. The passive partner engaging in anal sex, for example, is at far greater risk of contracting the virus than the active partner or those engaging in vaginal sex. This is because the rectum is easily traumatized and torn during such activity, providing easier access for HIV to enter the bloodstream. Oral sex is a less likely means of transmission, but cases have been known to occur. The virus can effectively be transmitted by transfusion of infected blood, via needle injuries, exposure of open wounds to infected body fluids, and perinatal transmission from infected mother to infant. But with all cases, the risk of infection has to do not only with how many viral particles are transmitted from one person to another but also with a wide variety of other factors we are only beginning to appreciate. For example, because of genetic and immunological reasons not yet entirely clear, it is entirely possible for someone to be exposed to HIV but not become infected at all.

HIV belongs to a rather interesting family of viruses called retrovirus. Unlike human cells whose genes consist of strands of DNA, retrovirus genes are composed of RNA, a molecule that humans (and, in fact, most living organisms) employ as a messenger from one part of the body to the other to carry out genetic orders. Like all viruses, HIV can replicate only inside the cells of its host, requiring it to come up with novel means of breaking and entering before commandeering the cells' machinery to reproduce thousands of copies of itself. As scientists have since discovered, HIV has managed to develop a superbly effective means of accomplishing this delicate task.

The primary target for the human immunodeficiency virus is a particular type of white blood cell called a $T_4$-helper or $CD_4$ lymphocyte. Like a lock and key, the virus binds to a molecule on the lymphocyte's surface, called the $CD_4$ receptor, which essentially opens the cell's door and allows the virus to gain entry. Once inside, HIV, a most greedy habitué, garnishees the use of an enzyme called reverse transcriptase that already exists in the host's lymphocytes. This enzyme converts the virus's RNA-based genes into the language of DNA, thus allowing it to be spliced into the host's genetic code. The result is that even after the virus has jumped to another part of the body, the infected cells are busy making viral copies on its behalf that continuously worsen the infection. The hijacked human cells, in essence, become HIV viral factories.

Physicians like to anthropomorphize diseases, giving their foes human qualities far beyond reality. I must admit, I readily subscribe to this quaint practice and have always been amazed by HIV's cunning powers. Think for a moment about its brilliance as an agent that exists merely to destroy its victims' ability to fight off the daily onslaught of microbes. HIV searches out and destroys a lynchpin of the human immune system: the $CD_4$ or helper lymphocyte cell that acts as an accelerator of the body's complex response against foreign invasions. Under the right circumstances, $T_4$-helper cells send out chemical messages to other lymphocytes urging them to prepare for battle, to find and surround the interloper in question, and ultimately to engulf, destroy, and remove it from the body. When infected by HIV, the lymphocyte's genetic machinery is used for expressly evil purposes and the helper cells are rendered all but useless. The greater the viral load, the more advanced the infection, the fewer the helper cells available. The results are always catastrophic, because without adequate numbers of these T-helper cells neither B-lymphocytes nor cytotoxic T-lymphocytes, other critical actors in the immune system, can function properly. Ultimately, the immune system is reduced to being a prestigious symphony orchestra forced to play without its first or second violin sections.

In most cases, the person with HIV rarely knows exactly when he or she was first infected. The earliest stage is often confused with a garden variety cold, perhaps a fever, or maybe simply fatigue. Some people might develop mild diarrhea or a headache, or notice that the lymph nodes in their neck or under their armpits are slightly swollen and painful. But HIV, like syphilis, quiets down for long stretches of time, allowing its host to declare premature victory under the false assumption that it was just a touch of what's going around. This dormant period can last for years, but physicians have only recently begun to appreciate that clinical latency does not equal disease latency. Like a shark, HIV never sleeps. Unchecked, the virus continues to replicate and insert itself into the host's genetic code, destroying more and more T-helper cells minute by minute, day by day, year by year.

Eventually, this viral domination of the T-cells inexorably progresses and the body becomes more susceptible to specific infections that healthy people knock out of their system with the same force that Babe Ruth used to bat baseballs out of Yankee Stadium. Strange and exotic organisms such as cryptococcus or toxoplasmosis—fungal threats to animals but rarely to healthy human beings—soon become potential nuclear attacks on the bodies of AIDS patients. A simple bout of herpes on the lips or mouth—what many people dismiss as a cold sore—can potentially go wildly out of control and destroy an AIDS patient's brain in a matter of days.

As just one small but graphic example of what immune-compromised people must contend with, let's consider a fungal infection called *Candida albicans* that is most commonly seen in babies. Infants develop

*Candida* for the same reason AIDS patients get it; their immune system has a difficult time fighting off the fungus. Most mothers and fathers know it as thrush because of the cottony white patches that appear in the baby's mouth and look like the fluffy breast of the eponymous bird. But babies outgrow this stage of immuno-immaturity while people with AIDS descend only deeper and deeper into an immune-deficient hell. Calling these more serious candidal infections something as chirpy and light as thrush is an insult. For AIDS patients, *Candida* is a raw, bloody, and painful assault of the mouth and throat that often finds its way down to the esophagus and stomach. I have seen many patients with this malady for whom the simple act of sipping water was an excruciating experience. One memorably described it as "drinking a glass of razor blades."

Later, HIV can attack the neurological system with results ranging from intermittent lightning bolts of pain traveling along the nerve fibers and difficulties in balance and walking, to a wretched form of dementia. The blood-clotting system can fail, making small cuts serious injuries, or the bone marrow can refuse to produce a steady supply of nourishing red blood cells. The liver and kidneys can shut down and fail to cleanse the blood of toxins, creating metabolic nightmares. Often, strange malignancies develop into a cancerous blitzkrieg, such as Kaposi's sarcoma, a skin cancer formerly seen only in elderly men of Mediterranean heritage, that when augmented by AIDS goes wildly out of control and attacks the gut, the lungs, and even the brain. Both human and animal variants of tuberculosis now loom as hostile and daily threats to their victims' well-being. Add to this litany the wasting of one's body, the loss of muscle mass and its resultant weakness, deadly bouts of an exotic form of pneumonia called *Pneumocystis carinii,* hourly episodes of vomiting and diarrhea, and you begin to get a picture of how ubiquitous, how multisystemic, how powerful HIV can be.

Even today with revolutionary advances in anti-retroviral therapy, the cocktail of drugs that block the replication of HIV at different points of its life cycle, the battle is far from over. To be sure, these medications have made the terrible muscle wasting, endless diarrhea, and episodes of pneumocystis pneumonia that American physicians routinely saw in AIDS patients during the 1980s and early 1990s relatively rare events. But these potent medications can also be accompanied by dozens of serious if not intolerable side effects and may be ineffective for many patients. A newly recognized problem, again a function of the innate cleverness of the virus, is HIV's ability to change its structure ever so slightly and become resistant to the drugs we have, making matters of long-term treatment far more complex and uncertain.[26] While these medications have improved the survival rate of patients with HIV disease significantly, they are not a cure—only a stay of execution. HIV remains a microbe that likes to win all of its battles unequivocally.

When the first cases of AIDS were described in 1981, four major groups of people were implicated: homosexuals, heroin users, hemophiliacs, and Haitians—the so-called 4-H Club. The unfortunate designation of these four groups helped to create a powerful association of sexuality, substance abuse, "bad blood," black skin, voodoo rituals, and prejudice, as well as more mundane biological factors of disease causation. The confusion, finger-pointing, and fear that characterized the early years of the epidemic were only exacerbated by the fact that no one had a clear idea of what actually caused AIDS or how it was transmitted.

Before 1984, when Robert Gallo at the U.S. National Cancer Institute and Luc Montagnier of the Institut Pasteur in Paris independently identified HIV as the cause of this crisis in contagion, doctors and public health officials had little choice but to apply the *Casablanca* method of infection control.[27] In the opening scene of the classic Humphrey Bogart film, after someone is murdered in cold blood, the police captain Louis utters the famous line: "Round up the usual suspects." This is, in essence, what epidemiologists must do when confronted with an infection they do not understand; they round up every usual pathogenic suspect—and quite a few unusual ones—that might be at the root of the problem. It is only well after the discovery of cause and effect that the dry trails begin to look foolish.

One epidemiological detour explored was the potential link of AIDS to a drug called amyl nitrate. This substance was once used by doctors to treat patients with cardiac chest pain, or angina, because of its ability to widen blood vessels narrowed by fatty plaques of cholesterol. Amyl nitrate was eventually abandoned as a prescription drug in the 1960s because its major side effect was severe headaches. A much more tolerable form, nitroglycerine, is well known to those with heart disease today. By the 1970s, amyl nitrate became a treasured recreational drug, particularly within the gay community, for its other effects, including a pleasant head rush, muscle relaxation, and the enhancement of orgasm. During the 1970s and 1980s you could purchase little bottles of the stuff, with brand names like Poppers, Rush, and Locker Room, at any adult bookstore or discotheque in the country. As a result of this connection, public health officials spent months analyzing the compositions and strengths of different brands of amyl nitrate, their chemical properties when mixed with the lubricants used to perform anal sex, how much was inhaled, and several other permutations that might explain the drug's relationship to AIDS. It took months for public health experts to establish that while the drug is hardly safe for recreational use, it had little to do with the transmission or spread of the human immunodeficiency virus.[28]

In this atmosphere of "round up the usual suspects," the results of the discovery of AIDS among Haitian immigrants living in New York and South Florida, and among Haitians themselves, became all too predictable. As early as 1980, unusual deaths due to opportunistic infections such as cryptococcus, toxoplasmosis, *Pneumocystis carinii,* and atypical tuberculosis were reported in Haiti. The overwhelming majority of these patients were subsequently diagnosed with AIDS. Several epidemiological studies of asymptomatic Haitian city dwellers conducted during this period estimated HIV seroprevalance rates between 5 and 9 percent. By March 1990, the Pan American Health Organization confirmed that there were 2,331 cases of AIDS in Haiti and predicted that a large number of Haitians who engaged in high-risk behaviors in the larger cities were probably exposed to the virus.[29]

One Haitian physician named Jean Pape tracked these early cases of AIDS with a devotion and intensity worth mention. Dr. Pape founded the Haitian Study Group on Kaposi's Sarcoma and Opportunistic Infections (GHESKIO), which consisted of thirteen doctors and researchers. His team treated hundreds of HIV/AIDS patients in Haiti, in addition to conducting a series of elegant studies on the clinical and epidemiological puzzle unfolding on Hispaniola.

Early on in the epidemic, Pape documented several important aspects of the Haitian AIDS story that were not always appreciated by his American colleagues. While initially the majority of his patients were men, as the epidemic progressed he diagnosed more and more women with AIDS. Moreover, the epicenter of the epidemic was in the city of Carrefour, a suburb south of Port-au-Prince well known for its sex trade. Many of Dr. Pape's first AIDS patients were linked to prostitutes, male and female, or to people who frequently traveled to North Africa, where they had sexual contacts. There was also a relatively high rate of blood transfusion–associated cases that may have been related to the common practice of impoverished Haitians selling their blood and plasma to blood banks. After an extensive review of autopsy records, the clinical histories of the patients seen and treated at the GHESKIO Clinic, and epidemiological surveys of newly infected Haitians, Pape and his colleagues concluded that HIV was a relative newcomer to the island.[30]

Unfortunately, the well-documented investigations that Pape and his colleagues published in prominent American peer-reviewed medical journals were discounted by a large number of physicians practicing in the United States. Many American doctors publicly and arrogantly wondered if AIDS had existed in Haiti long before these reports but was simply overlooked by the physicians practicing there. The clear message was that Haitian doctors were not as well trained as their American counterparts and their diagnoses were not to be trusted. Other American physicians insisted that if AIDS did not originate in Haiti, it certainly predated its appearance in the United States. To make matters worse, some even proposed theories that AIDS stemmed from "bizarre voodoo practices and blood-drinking rituals" on Haiti, and that Haitian immigrants threatened to import more cases of the disease into the United States.[31] These biases were officially codified into medical dogma on March 23, 1983, when the United States Centers for Disease Control (CDC) defined Haitians as one of the four high-risk groups for AIDS.[32]

Most Haitian physicians objected strongly to these classifications and urged instead that the CDC warn Americans against the specific behaviors that made *all* human beings at risk for infection. In July 1983, Dr. Jean Claude Compas, the vice president of the Association of Haitian Physicians Abroad and co-chairman of the Haitian Coalition on AIDS, angrily testified before a U.S. congressional committee: "Most of the data used by the CDC and other health authorities were gathered by hospital-based physicians with no knowledge of French or Creole and who have admitted a complete ignorance of Haitian culture." Dr. Compas reminded his audience of the taboos against homosexuality in Haitian culture that might prevent a patient from discussing such sensitive issues with a physician he neither knew nor trusted. A colleague who joined him in the committee chamber, Dr. Robert Augusta, made the critical if ahistoric observation: "In the annals of medicine, this categorization of a nationality as a group at risk is unique."[33]

Casting the epidemiological net as widely as possible is common to the initial phase of virtually every public health crisis. But such medical detective work often has negative consequences for those labeled contagious. This was particularly true during the early years of the AIDS epidemic when there were no clear causal definitions or calibration of the risk factors for contracting the disease. In the eyes of most Americans, being labeled as a member of a "risk group" was synonymous with being both a carrier of AIDS and a public health threat.[34] Consequently, the net cast to contain AIDS stigmatized healthy Haitian immigrants living legally in the United States just as it did healthy members of the gay community.[35]

In Brooklyn and Manhattan, there were numerous reports of Haitian schoolchildren being beaten up and ostracized by their native-born American peers to prevent them from "infecting the neighborhood." Similarly, several grocery stores refused to serve Haitian customers for fear that they might spread AIDS to other customers.[36] In Florida, where the Haitian presence was even greater, businesses employing Haitians were bombarded with vicious hate mail warning them to avoid the immigrants at all costs, such as the following flyer reprinted in the *Miami Herald*:

> On Tuesday, July 19th [1983] we are mailing 6000 of the below notices to all hotels, motels, and restaurants in South Florida: "Tourists and business people are avoiding the South Florida area because of the plague of AIDS, hepatitis, and TB spread by the criminal, illegal aliens of Haitian origin. If you employ a Haitian, discharge him as soon as you receive this letter. Help South Florida."[37]

The Haitian community, of course, objected vigorously. Between 1983 and 1986, Haitian community activists organized on several fronts to protest their being classified en masse as a high-risk AIDS group. These activities included lobbying public health organizations, writing letters to newspapers and medical journals about the flawed epidemiological reports that singled out Haitians, initiating legal proceedings, and holding large public rallies to publicize their cause.

One small victory that emerged from these protests occurred in the summer of 1983 when the New York City Health Department removed Haitians from its official list of AIDS "high-risk groups" even though they continued to be classified as "high-risk" by the U.S. Centers for Disease Control for another two years. Nevertheless, for the Haitian community, the social damage had already been done, and it would require far greater measures than the mere revision of local health regulations or federal circulars to undo it. In the minds of the majority of Americans, AIDS was as firmly associated with Haitians as it was with the other "high-risk groups." As Dr. Jean Claude Compas, now representing the Haitian Medical Association of New York, commented: "After all the wild theories of voodoo rites and genetic predispositions were aired and dispelled, and the slipshod scientific investigations were brought to light, the public perception of the problem has remained the same—that if Haitians have AIDS, it is simply because they are Haitian."[38]

Perhaps the public health edict that most roiled the Haitian-American community was the ban against their donating blood in the United States. Long after the U.S. Public Health Service and the CDC lifted its "high-risk" designation of Haitians, the U.S. Food and Drug Administration (which has final jurisdiction over blood supply issues) kept its order in place. The intention of this recommendation, of course, was to take absolutely no chances with possible infection of the blood supply. The FDA insisted that it was working on a principle of "better safe than sorry." Initially, it barred Haitians who arrived in the United States *after* 1977 from donating blood. On February 5, 1990, however, the FDA handed down a new ruling prohibiting *all* Haitians from doing so.

Even with the best of epidemic control intentions, the FDA ban that exclusively targeted Haitians is difficult to comprehend. As one editorialist for the *Boston Globe* argued, if the FDA was justifying a public health need to ban blood donations based purely on geographical risk, it should have imposed one on San Franciscans, residents of a city where, according to the CDC, the AIDS case rate in 1989 was 114.5 per 100,000 people. Bans would also be more prudent in San Juan, Puerto Rico, where the case rate was 86.8 per 100,000 residents, New York City (69.4 per 100,000), or Boston (58.1 per 100,000). In comparison, in 1989, the AIDS case rate in Haiti was actually less than 12 per 100,000.[39]

This ruling also ignored the Haitian cultural belief that an accusation of "dirty blood" (*san sal*) is a highly insulting assessment of one's character or morality. The declaration means that one's "bad deeds are the inevitable results of bad blood." In essence, the FDA's blood donation ban was an official proclamation that *all* Haitians had *san sal*.[40] Consequently, many Haitian immigrants living in the United States, who were turned away for performing a selfless and charitable act, perceived the FDA's ruling as remarkably offensive if not sinister.

The prognosis of which event will drive a particular community to its strongest response is a difficult enterprise. Sometimes an inflammatory spark is nothing more than a brief moment of flash and light that all too quickly fades into darkness. At other historical moments the spark incites a full-fledged flame. The FDA ruling on Haitian blood donations instigated the latter type of response: on March 7, 1990, over five thousand Haitian Americans picketed the Miami FDA office, an act of civil disobedience that halted traffic at Miami International Airport for hours. Their picket signs declared in blood red paint: "FDA = Federal Discrimination Agency."[41]

A few weeks later, on April 20, in New York City, the Haitians' outrage at the blood ban resulted in a massive rally. More than 50,000 people marched across the Brooklyn Bridge to City Hall to protest the FDA's discriminatory edict, forcing the police to close this fabled pathway across the East River. Joining the Haitians were motion picture actors Susan Sarandon and Tim Robbins, the Reverend Jesse Jackson, the newly elected mayor of New York, David Dinkins, and a huge throng of white and African-American supporters. The Haitian-American newspaper *Haiti-Progrès* described the protest as a stunning event whose magnitude "had not been seen in New York since the 1968 funeral of Martin Luther King."[42] Almost a week after the march, a headline boldly published in the *New York Daily News* nicely captured the Haitian-American community's impression of the march: "Haitians Surprised, Too."[43]

Shortly after the New York City protest, the FDA formed an advisory committee to reconsider the ruling, and within a week the group recommended that donor bans based on geographic or national origin end. Not everyone agreed. For example, the *New York Times*, which had generally been sympathetic to the Haitian cause, editorialized a strong condemnation of the move: "the FDA needs to think more carefully before accepting its committee's advice. Preventing discrimination is a high priority. Keeping the blood supply free of deadly disease and ensuring adequate supplies surely ranks even higher."[44] However, the majority of American public health experts argued the geographical ban was causing more harm than good. By 1990, developments such as identifying the etiologic agent, HIV, the discovery of a blood test to determine if someone had actually been exposed to the virus, and common sense encouraged a policy whereby *all* blood donations or products would be scrutinized for HIV regardless of the donor's geographic origins.

In December 1990, after a series of marches across the United States, culminating with one that began on the steps of the U.S. Capitol and ended at the front door of the FDA headquarters in Rockville, Mary-

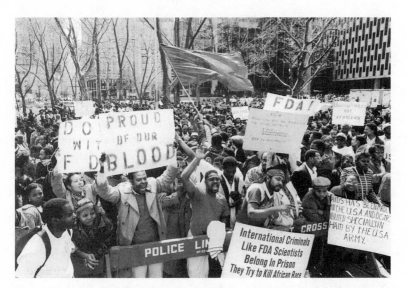

*More than 50,000 Haitian immigrants and supporters partic-
ipated in an AIDS rally in New York City on April 20, 1990.*

land, the FDA formally removed Haitians from its list of banned blood
donors. Beyond the stigma of AIDS, the color of their skin, or the status
of immigrant, it was the issue of blood that most mobilized the Haitian-
American community. More than a decade later, many still recall "April
20," or "the March," as a pivotal event in their history. As the Haitian-
American journalist Barbara Sanon explained, the march "was a defining
moment for Haitians, a rekindling of resistance that dates back to their
bloody overthrow of French slave owners in 1804. Those of us there that
day will never forget how our *fyète ayisyen* (Haitian pride) shook the
Brooklyn Bridge, cleansing our reputation and keeping our blood
intact—if still boiling."[45]

There are nine counties, or *départements,* in Haiti, and a popular saying among Haitians is that the United States is Haiti's "tenth
*département.*"[46] Long before HIV made its way to Haiti's shores, the
country was plagued by enough social problems to inspire thousands of
Haitians to leave. As Jean-Bertrand Aristide, Haiti's first democratically
elected president in 1990, explained: "Haiti is the parish of the poor. In

Haiti, it is not enough to heal wounds, for every day another wound opens up."[47] But in the months following the 1991 coup that deposed Aristide, the floodgates controlling emigration toppled and thousands of Haitians headed toward the United States. In response to this crisis, President George H. W. Bush ordered the Coast Guard to intercept their boats at sea and to take them to the U.S. naval base at Guantánamo Bay, Cuba, for questioning about their eligibility for political asylum. More than 40,000 Haitian refugees were intercepted at sea and approximately 75 percent of them were ultimately returned to Haiti.

Guantánamo Naval Base, on the southern tip of Cuba, is one of the strangest military installations in the world. The base overlooks Guantánamo Bay and is almost equidistant between Jamaica and Haiti. The United States has leased this plot of land from Cuba since 1903 in an ironclad agreement that neither Fidel Castro nor the Cold War could revoke. Between 1991 and 1993, 12,000 Haitians who were deemed most likely to be granted asylum status by the U.S. Immigration and Naturalization Service were detained on Guantánamo. Of these, more than 11,000 were ultimately allowed to enter the United States as political asylees. All 12,000 refugees were tested for HIV as part of the U.S. immigration policy begun in 1986. About 200 tested positive, including Tomás, and they—and 55 of their immediate relatives—stayed on Guantánamo, in quarantine, for almost two years.

By mid-1992, however, it was clear that this approach was not doing enough to stem the tide of Haitian boat people. Consequently, on May 24, 1992, President Bush redoubled his efforts by ordering a complete blockade of Haiti and directing the Coast Guard to immediately return all refugees to Haiti—no questions asked—with the suggestion that those seeking political asylum begin the process at the U.S. Embassy in Port-au-Prince.[48] A year later, on June 21, 1993, the U.S. Supreme Court ruled 8–1 to allow the Clinton administration to continue halting Haitian refugees on the high seas and forcibly sending them back to their homeland. For those fleeing the Haitian military, this order of return was essentially a death sentence.[49]

Finding reliable historical documentation about the Guantánamo refugee camp is difficult because neither the captors nor the captives want to talk much about it. However, some details, though skewed, have been recorded. One U.S. Navy sailor stationed at "Gitmo" in the early 1990s posted a website on the Internet entitled "God and Country Presents GTMO's Haitian Invasion: The Day We Bit Off a Little More Than We Could Chew." Complete with photographs of the United States Coast Guard cutters bringing Haitian refugees to the base and the "tent city" set up on an airstrip, his recollections of how "these would-be illegal immigrants were intercepted and sent to <u>our</u> [his underline] island home" are interesting, to say the least:

> I remember seeing the first Coast Guard cutters arrive. They were moored out in the bay for days before being allowed to dock at Fleet Landing. Many of us drove up to McCalla Hill with binoculars in hand to get a better look at what was going on. No one was really telling us anything. First one ship and then another. A corpsman-chief friend, who had to go out there and assess their health returned with wild stories of disease, sexual diviance [*sic*], homosexuality and the strange way they let nature call.[50]

Armed with a camera, a video recorder, and a pad of government-issued paper, the sailor worried about "what we would do with all of the Haitian's [*sic*] infected with AIDS." Woven throughout his memoir is a ribbon of resentment against the Haitians who ruined a favorite strip of beach where he would "drag-race my pick-em-up truck, run my weiny [*sic*] dog, and fly kites." He also displays a common brand of American myopia that assumes wherever we plant the "Stars and Stripes" is "home," even if it is flown above a foreign land.

The airstrip, McCalla Airfield, became the site of thousands of tents surrounded by a threatening barrier of razor-sharp barbed wire and armed military guards keeping careful watch. Again, the sailor's observations:

> The press called McCalla's tent cities "Confinement Camps" and to a certain extent they were right. However, there were many good reasons, including 7,000 [American] residents of Guantanamo Bay, in which my wife and I were part of. We barely had the accommodations, food and water for our population let alone 12,000 more. The majority of Haitians couldn't communicate in English, were uneducated and unskilled. Many of the Haitians were infected with AIDS, Hepatitis, Malaria and other forms of communicable diseases. The threats to GTMO resident's [*sic*] peace, health, and safety were many. The only way to maintain control of an increasingly chaotic situation was limit the movement of these migrants.[51]

The sailor also chastised the Haitians for being too "primitive" to use the toilet facilities provided for them and therefore posing another health risk to U.S. citizens:

> Most were set in their ways and just let nature take its course when ever and where ever [*sic*] they pleased. With thousands of Haitians in such a confined area—this wasn't healthy at all. For the hard core dumpers, we at least convinced them to crap on paper plates so that it could be cleaned up more easily.[52]

In actuality, the American sailor exaggerated his argument on many points, particularly in his assessment of the health status of the incarcerated Haitians and the naval base's ability to get all the food and provisions it required to feed the military personnel. Moreover, the sanitary amenities provided for the 12,000 Haitians by their American hosts consisted of a dozen Port-a-Potties. It was hardly "primitive behavior" for the refugees to avoid these stinking, overflowing privies. But the sailor's recollections *do* accurately reflect the feelings and resentments many Americans had toward the Haitian refugees during this period.[53]

For those living behind the barbed wire, of course, the perspective was markedly different. Dr. Paul Farmer, a physician and medical anthropologist at Harvard Medical School, conducted a number of interviews with Guantánamo inmates during this period. One of his subjects, a woman named Yolanda Jean, eloquently described the harsh realities of life in the Haitian refugee camp:

> We were in a space cordoned off with barbed wire. Wherever they put you, you were meant to stay right there; there was no place to move. The latrines were brimming over. There was never any cool water to drink, to wet our lips. There was only water in a cistern, boiling in the hot sun. When you drank it, it gave you diarrhea. . . . Rats crawled over us at night. . . . When you saw these things, we thought, it's not possible, it can't go on like this. We're humans, just like everyone else.[54]

Eventually the tents were replaced by makeshift barracks, but the roofs were leaky and required patching with plastic garbage bags. A significant number of the inmates were children. One infant, who was not HIV-positive, died of pneumonia, an infection that could have been treated successfully in the United States. Other children incurred injuries and

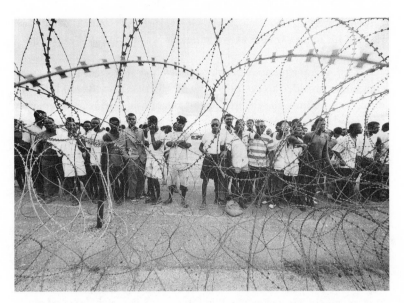

*Scores of Haitian refugee men stand behind a razor-wire enclosed*
*camp at Guantánamo Bay Naval Base, December 29, 1991.*

lacerations from playing too close to the barbed-wire fence. There were
also reports of frequent beatings, destruction of personal property, and
other forms of brutality.[55] These harsh conditions led to hunger strikes,
suicide attempts, and protests, including an attempt by sixty-three
Haitians to set fire to one of the plywood barracks in August 1993. But all
of the refugees' demands to be sent back to Haiti or some other location,
no matter how incendiary, angry, or eloquent, were denied.[56]

The experiences of the HIV-positive prisoners, isolated in a special
section called Camp Bulkeley, were even worse. Here Tomás was confined with the other HIV-positive detainees and their relatives. In 1992
medical science had relatively few laboratory markers to assess how
much damage the virus had done to a patient's immune system beyond
the T-lymphocyte count. During most of his stay on Guantánamo,
Tomás's T-count was well above 700, and, consequently, he did not need
to take anti-retroviral medication. Toward the end of his internment at
Camp Bulkeley, however, Tomás's T-cell count dipped below 500, which
represented the clinical indication for physicians to prescribe anti-

retroviral medications such as AZT (zidovudine). Tomás's perception was that his imprisonment at Guantánamo was responsible for the progression of his disease.

Indeed, many egregious problems prevented adequate medical care from being provided to the prisoners on Guantánamo. Beyond the differences of culture, the doctor-patient relationship, which sits squarely on a foundation of trust and open dialogue, was severely perverted, if not outright destroyed. This, undoubtedly, had a negative effect on the health of the inmates, who had little confidence in their doctors' judgment and often ignored their medical recommendations. What health care was provided to the Haitians was done in an atmosphere of brazen disrespect. If a refugee refused to submit to a medical examination on a particular day, a group of military police—gloved, masked, and "protected"—would physically lift him up and take him to the base clinic. Once there, they would pin their bodies against him so that the corpsman could quickly place a tourniquet around his arm, search for a vein, and draw a few vials of blood for the laboratory. Similarly, several women complained about unexplained and forcible injections that turned out to be the birth-control agent Depo-Provera. Among the side effects of these injections were a disruption of many of the women's menstrual cycles, occasional periods of heavy vaginal bleeding, and a deep sense of outrage. The medical team at Guantánamo explained that the contraceptive measures were medically indicated because of the risks to both an HIV-positive woman who became pregnant and her unborn child. Such forcible approaches to health care would be condemned by any civilized country, and most medical ethicists and lawyers would classify these actions as felonious assault.[57]

Haitian activists and others made repeated pleas to the U.S. government to release the HIV-positive Haitians or at least provide real humanitarian aid, but little was done. The comments of President Bush's INS spokesman, Duke Austin, best reflected the U.S. government's attitude at the time. He refused to acknowledge the moral, ethical, and legal repercussions of imprisoning HIV-positive refugees. "They're gonna die anyway, right?" he asked a crowd of scribbling journalists just before Christmas in 1992.[58] Equally, if not more insensitive, when a hypothetical question was raised a few months later over what the government's policy ought to be for a child dying of AIDS whose last wish was to visit Disneyland, Congressman Tom DeLay (R-Texas) callously replied, "Let them go to Disneyland in France. You've got to be hard in situations like this."[59]

At the same time, public health experts began writing memoranda to officials in the U.S. Justice Department about the grave public health dangers that might develop because of the Haitian internment policy. For example, Dr. Paul V. Effler of the CDC wrote: "It is common sense, I think, to realize that concentrating people known to have an infection that causes immunosuppression in a tent city is a potential health disaster." Similarly, Dr. James Mason, assistant secretary of health and chief of the United States Public Health Service, repeatedly expressed serious concerns about the "substantial risks" for "uncontrolled, sustained transmission of infectious diseases" among those infected with HIV and others living at the camp.[60]

Perhaps the crux of "the Guantánamo problem" was the widespread fear among many Americans that opening the door even a bit to the Haitians was akin to an engraved invitation for HIV-positive immigrants from around the world to settle in the United States. Consider a CNN/*Time* poll taken in early February 1993 that asked the question "Should the United States allow foreigners who have the AIDS virus to enter?" Of those polled, 71 percent said "no," 22 percent "yes," and the remaining 7 percent were undecided. Not surprisingly, the most common reason offered for such a ban was one that immigration restrictionists have used since at least the beginning of the twentieth century: the threat of economic ruin posed by caring for sickly newcomers. As Dan Stein, the executive director of the Federation for American Immigration Reform, warned, "Our medical care, social services net and free public education are a magnet for immigrants."[61]

On February 17, 1993, Senator Don Nickles (R-Oklahoma) introduced an amendment to a bill that would extend the ban on HIV-positive immigrants. Nickles insisted that his motivations had nothing to do with either fear or homophobia. Instead, his amendment was based purely out of concern that allowing HIV-infected immigrants to enter would overwhelm the American health care system, "jeopardize the lives of countless Americans," and "cost the U.S. taxpayers millions of dollars."[62] The American Medical Association supported this position, urging a continuation of the ban because "we do not need any more AIDS patients."[63] The bill passed the Senate overwhelmingly, 76–23, and a few weeks later with an even larger show of support in the House of Representatives. Perhaps no member of Congress expressed the rationale behind it more clearly than Congressman Robert Dornan (R-California):

What we are talking about is letting in people into this country in their young years—look at the profile of Haitians—in their young years, what liberals call raging hormone-sexually active years into this country with a communicable venereal disease that is always fatal. . . . It is a Haitian problem. . . . But we cannot let in people with a venereal disease that is communicable. That would kill Americans, and it is stupid.[64]

On June 10, 1993, President Bill Clinton signed into law the National Institutes of Health Revitalization Act. In its many pages and among the legalistic maze of clauses was an amendment to the Immigration and Nationality Act of 1988 that specifically included infection with HIV as a legitimate reason to bar an alien's entry into the United States. Only a few years earlier, then-candidate Clinton ran on a platform pledging to remove or fight bans against a disease that was anything but casual in its transmission.[65] But even though the gates of immigration were now effectively closed to all newcomers infected with HIV, the Haitian refugee problem on Guantánamo remained and it demanded a more humane form of resolution than simply waiting for those people to die.

Coincident with the legislative and executive proceedings over HIV and immigration, a group of Haitian immigrants and attorneys from the American Civil Liberties Union and the National Coalition for Haitian Refugees filed a lawsuit against the Immigration and Naturalization Service and the U.S. naval base at Guantánamo for their actions against the HIV-positive Haitian refugees. The suit was filed in Brooklyn, New York, before the Eastern District of the United States District Court because one of the plaintiffs lived in Brooklyn's Haitian community. It came to trial in late February 1993.

At the trial, one physician stationed at Guantánamo testified he had repeatedly recommended medical evacuations for those deemed most advanced in their disease, but his requests were routinely ignored. Even some of the government lawyers admitted that the Haitians with "full-blown AIDS" were not receiving sufficient treatment at Guantánamo. As a result of these testimonies, the U.S. district judge, Sterling Johnson Jr., ordered that those medically evaluated with AIDS (approximately forty refugees) be immediately transferred to the closest place where they could receive adequate care other than Haiti, "to prevent any loss of life." On March 27, they were flown to Miami for treatment.[66] Nevertheless, the trial continued until mid-June in order to address the final destination of the other two hundred HIV-positive detainees and their family members.

Judge Johnson was new to the role he found himself playing. Only recently appointed to the bench, he had spent most of his career as the special narcotics prosecutor for New York City. Yet he demonstrated that the time spent wearing a judicial robe was less important than a healthy common sense and conscience when deliberating cases like this one. After listening carefully to two very different sides of the same story, on June 8, Johnson announced in a somewhat acerbic opinion that he was not at all impressed by the U.S. government's case and ordered the release of the HIV-positive Haitians:

> Although the defendants euphemistically refer to its Guantánamo operation as a "humanitarian camp," the facts disclose that it is nothing more than an HIV prison camp presenting potential public health risks to Haitians held there. The Haitians' plight is a tragedy of immense proportions and their continued detainment is totally unacceptable to this Court.[67]

Outside the courtroom, U.S. Justice officials carped about Judge Johnson's "expansive" views of the rights of immigrants "who came into American hands purely out of our own humanitarian impulses to rescue them at sea." But a lawyer for the Center for Constitutional Reform, Michael Ratner, who worked on behalf of the Haitians, provided a far more measured perspective: "I don't think of this as winning, just as ending an ordeal for people who may have spent a significant part of their remaining lives in a prison camp."[68]

Rather than appeal the decision, the U.S. government took the necessary steps to close Camp Bulkeley at Guantánamo. On June 12 the remaining Haitians interned there were given a new set of clothes, instructed to pack their belongings if they had any, and flown to Miami International Airport via a military cargo transport plane. In Miami the bedraggled and tired refugees were met by representatives of the local Haitian community who, like many an immigrant group before them, were prepared to help the newcomers adjust to their new lives. Unlike the multitude of predecessors, however, these refugees had to bear the oppressive stigma of being infected with HIV.

At the airport gate, eager to greet his countrymen, was Frantz Lieuman. A thirty-two-year-old native of Port-au-Prince, Frantz spent ten months on Guantánamo, but because his disease was so advanced he was one of the refugees evacuated by Judge Johnson's order at the end of March 1993. Now on several medications but medically stable, Frantz heartily endorsed Judge Johnson's decision: "Haiti is a prison and so is Guantánamo. In both places, the military is in charge and no one has any rights."[69]

Many of the newly released Haitians complained to the reporters covering their arrival that the HIV diagnoses were merely a ploy to keep them out of the United States and insisted that they were healthy. For example, before boarding the military plane to join his relatives in Miami, Nelson Armel remarked: "They tell me that I have the virus but they offer no proof. The first thing I am going to do is see a doctor and find out the truth." Another refugee, Joseph-Marie Rosit, commented bitterly, "If we have the virus, why haven't they given us any medicine for it?"[70] When considering the overwhelming difficulties these refugees endured in the form of physical threats and the dangerous escape from Haiti, imprisonment on Guantánamo, and, of course, the unkindest cut of all, their discovery of being infected with HIV, declarations of denial seem quite reasonable. This defense mechanism was an essential element of their survival—which had been the whole point of their flight.

Long after the turmoil of the military coup, the murders, and the dramatic escape attempts of thousands of Haitians, long after the protest marches and the impassioned speeches by Hollywood actors, rock stars, and politicians to do something about the Haitians' plight, long after their captivity on Guantánamo and the diagnosis of HIV infection in a tiny fraction of the inmates, long after the short-lived restoration of a democratically elected government in Haiti and the U.S. Supreme Court's ruling that upheld the INS policy of returning all subsequent Haitians found at sea, there were—as there always are in the life of a person with a serious illness—the daily depressing, demeaning, and often humiliating realities of disease.

Most of the Haitians discovered to have HIV on Guantánamo ultimately settled in Miami and Brooklyn. But their new lives in the United States remained intensely difficult, if not surreal. Tomás was one of the Guantánamo inmates who arrived in Brooklyn in the late summer of 1993, and by the following year his condition developed into full-blown AIDS. With assistance from some charitable aid agencies and food stamps, he eked out a precarious existence in a studio apartment in the Flatbush section of Brooklyn. He soon became bored and tired of keeping track of the almost fifty pills he took at precise times each day and an unproductive routine of visits to busy doctors, harried social workers, and overworked attorneys all with overflowing case loads. On many days, Tomás wandered the streets and occasionally mustered the energy for a visit to Manhattan. During these months he rarely discussed his HIV status with others, but the painful isolation that marked his days ravaged his mind every bit as effectively as the HIV virus took over his immune system.

By early 1995, Tomás was in his mid-thirties but looked like an old man. His weight was little more than half of what it was before leaving Haiti. He appeared drawn, exhausted, and exhibited a wobbly and laborious gait whenever he tried to walk. Tomás was deathly ill. He was drinking a lot of beer and wine to pass the day, mostly to numb his senses to the horrors of his present and future, despite repeated warnings that alcohol had the potential to worsen his disease and cause other health problems. He became incontinent, which prevented him from even the occasional luxury of going out for a brief walk because he would immediately have to run back to his apartment to use the toilet. No one had much to offer this proud man whose ambition was once to open a small grocery store in his village and, perhaps, earn enough to get to America. While he certainly did come to the United States, it was on terms no one would have agreed to. Tomás died, alone in his tiny apartment, on a cold, bleak February day in 1995. Several days later his landlady let herself into his apartment because he had not paid his rent and she was wondering if something might have happened to him. She was appalled by the stench of death and the spectacle of a six-foot-four-inch corpse that weighed little more than 105 pounds. Only a priest and his social worker attended Tomás's funeral at a tiny church in Brooklyn.

A few years later, in 1998, the *New York Times* published a story about the forgotten plight of the HIV-positive Haitians. One survivor, Amos Dacy, who also settled in Brooklyn, remarked: "I think that if I had stayed in Haiti, I would have been killed. Now I wonder if it's worse to die alone." Another refugee, who did not want to give his name to the reporter, said: "I'm constantly reminded that I'm not home. When I walk down the street, I don't know when they're going to come and send me back so I'm always on edge."[71]

Tomás, at least, does not have to worry about asylum applications, green cards, or doctors' appointments. Perhaps, if he could have freed himself from the bondage of his fearsome fate, he might have been able to offer some sympathetic advice to Amos about the ordeal of dying alone in a foreign land. In any case, the tragic deaths of the HIV-positive

Haitians once interned on Guantánamo cannot silence the screaming facts of this ongoing epidemic. At the end of 2003, the World Health Organization estimated that 40 million people are living in the world with HIV. This breaks down to about one in every 100 adults. Seventy percent of the world's HIV-positive population live in sub-Saharan Africa, where one of every four people is HIV-positive, and 17 percent live in South and Southeast Asia.

Today, AIDS is the fourth leading killer in the world, and it is steadily gaining ground, especially in the developing world, where 95 percent of all new infections are diagnosed. Every day approximately 15,000 people are infected with HIV and about half of them are between the ages of fifteen and twenty-four years. Over 12 million young people around the world were infected and an estimated 14 million children younger than fifteen lost their mother or both parents to AIDS at the end of 2002.[72] The future appears even bleaker. Over the next decade, the next wave of AIDS is likely to be centered in China, Ethiopia, India, Nigeria, and Russia, where more than 40 percent of the world's population live, and public health experts predict a rise from 14 to 23 million HIV-infected people to 50 to 75 million. Such a massive increase in disease has prompted the U.S. Central Intelligence Agency to classify AIDS as one of the greatest potential security threats facing these regions and the United States in the years to come. Equally disturbing, by 2020, the United Nations has forecast that AIDS will claim the lives of at least an additional 65 million people, more than three times the number of deaths during the first twenty years of the epidemic, "unless more countries vastly expand their prevention programs."[73] There are many powerful forces that continue to feed this epidemic, including poverty, lifestyle behaviors, international travel, and discrimination. But these are only some of the major obstacles to effective HIV/AIDS prevention and care that we must surmount. Inertia, the steadfast failure to act definitively in the face of a crisis, remains the most difficult trend to reverse in this worldwide pandemic.

# SIX

# Sounding the Cholera Alarm in Detroit

A lot of the doctors who have come to visit us lately have just assumed we were "sick" or "diseased" as opposed to simply being from a different country. There is a difference, you know?

—ABRAHAM, a sixteen-year-old refugee from
Ethiopia living at Freedom House in Detroit

O nly a stone's throw from the Ambassador Bridge, a thoroughfare that spans the international border between the United States (Detroit, Michigan) and Canada (Windsor, Ontario) stands a century-old ramshackle former convent on the grounds of Detroit's oldest Catholic church, St. Anne's. Today, the red brick building, with its forty bedrooms, two bathrooms, kitchen, some offices, and a few common areas, serves as a hostel for refugees who come to the United States seeking asylum. It is aptly named Freedom House and is situated on a barren stretch of land near Detroit's "Mexican Village." Along with the Ambassador Bridge, the church is one of two identifiable landmarks in a desolate neighborhood inhabited primarily by outdated industrial buildings, struggling Mexican immigrants, and, as the 1980s progressed and the drug trade swept into this portion of the Motor City, crack houses.

Downtown Detroit was never much to brag about. Even before the devastating race riots of the 1960s and the urban white flight, this city was hardly a destination for the chic metropolitan. For more than a century, Detroit had been a factory town—perhaps the largest factory town in the history of humankind, thanks to our insatiable thirst for bigger and faster automobiles—situated on a thin wisp of a river, the Detroit. Today, greater metropolitan Detroit is comprised of many cities and might be best described as a large doughnut of settlements with the hole being the central city itself surrounded by dozens of suburbs of varying ethnic and socioeconomic mixes.

Long before urban decay, however, came the construction of deeply recessed concrete expressways that not only provided rapid exits out of the city but also sliced up the neighborhoods that remained. For example, Freedom House is about fifteen blocks from downtown's modest collection of office buildings, hotels, and, lately, new sports complexes and gambling casinos. But in order to get there, one must traverse a pedestrian bridge across the threatening valley created by a six-lane freeway. Just a bit to the west, north, and east are more vacant lots and abandoned buildings than you are likely to see in the center of any other American city. Detroit once boasted the most square feet of living space per resident in the form of freestanding homes, but today many of its residential neighborhoods are in a poor state of health, if not outright dead.[1] Over the past few decades, however, Detroit has become a stop on the "underground railroad" of our era; it is a popular way station for many refugees and immigrants, who arrive with the intention of crossing still another international border—to Canada.[2]

At any given time, twenty-five to forty different nations are represented at Freedom House, making every interaction a linguistic and cultural challenge. The residents' travel routes vary, but the predominant means of transportation are jumbo jets. Large airports, such as John F. Kennedy in New York, O'Hare in Chicago, Miami International, and Los Angeles International, are as permanently implanted in the minds of today's most recent immigrants as Ellis Island was for so many newcomers a century ago.[3]

In the fall of 1997, I was asked to volunteer some time at Freedom House by its then executive director, a tall, blond-haired, and energetic woman named Lynne Partington. Her commitment and devotion to her immigrant clients was as noble, if far more unsung, than the social workers who staffed the legendary settlement houses during the first great wave of immigration, like the Henry Street House in New York City[4] or Hull House in Chicago.[5] But in addition to the complexities of assimilation and social hostilities that the indefatigable Lillian Wald and Jane Addams tackled, Partington wrestled with a portfolio of problems accompanying today's immigrants that might have shocked her predecessors: harrowing escapes from political turmoil, physical violence, and death in war-torn nations; drug and alcohol abuse; few social support networks or relatives living in the United States; and a host of legal, economic, psychiatric, and medical problems. Like those who took care of the needs of past generations of immigrants, the staff at Freedom House had pitifully little money or professional resources to aid their cause. But none of these deficits were powerful enough to deter them. When standing in Lynne's office, one could almost hear her desk groan under the weight of the thick files and problem lists—each one representing a different resident—that were stacked in neat piles.

While eager to help, I had relatively few illusions that either the staff or residents were interested in me because of the years I had spent in libraries or book-lined seminar rooms writing and arguing about the immigration experience. No high-flown academic theories were needed in this living, breathing social laboratory. Instead, I was being recruited because of my medical license and willingness to provide some basic (and free) medical care for the children and adults who found their disrupted lives now unfolding at Freedom House.

I agreed to come weekly, every Friday afternoon, and my first "house call" was on a bleak, cold day in January 1998. I arrived several minutes before the appointed noon hour and decided to wander about the church grounds. There's a frigid chill to Michigan winters that descends shortly after Christmas and remains well into spring, hurting one's chest when drawing in air as if the bronchi and bronchioles were freezing and snapping with each breath. It is not the white, fluffy snowy scenes of greeting cards. Instead, southeastern Michigan is encased in a gray, sunless, frozen stretch of time lasting months. Such weather is vexing enough for those of us who have lived for years in this part of the world. One can only imagine what a harsh welcome it must be to those immigrants who arrived from locations if not more politically or economically stable, at least warmer.

Not far from Freedom House there is a bronze historical marker commemorating St. Anne's and its significance to Detroit. On July 24, 1701, Antoine de la Mothe Cadillac led a party of two hundred French settlers onto the sandy banks of the Detroit River to found Ville d'étroit, "the city on the narrow strait."[6] Within two days, they founded St. Anne's Catholic Church.[7] Almost a century later, the parish hired a remarkable Jesuit priest named Gabriel Richard (1767–1832). Among his many accomplishments, Richard represented the Michigan Territory in the United States Congress from 1823 to 1825, founded Michigan's first newspaper, *The Michigan Essay and Impartial Observer*, and, along with two other territorial settlers, the institution that ultimately became the University of Michigan.[8] The marker also describes how the good father died a miserable death during the first cholera epidemic in American history—a worldwide pandemic that was thought to have crossed the Atlantic Ocean in the bodies of immigrants—on September 13, 1832. A pastor in the fullest sense of the word, Father Richard contracted the infection during his round-the-clock visits to the ill and dying.[9]

Inside Freedom House, the vestibule was a stark sight: Lynne's office, once the house's front parlor, was to the left, and a smaller office overflowing with desks and chairs was to the right. Dominating the entranceway was a large and somewhat unstable-appearing staircase that sagged in the middle of each step as if an elephant had just climbed it and left an imprint. Off to the side of the steps was a pay phone with phone numbers written on the wall surrounding it. Front and center in the vestibule was an informal greeting committee of fifteen residents. Some were from Africa, a few from the Middle East, more were from Central and South America. Despite the ethnicity many wore on their faces, their clothes were primarily drawn from the collection box. Hence the odd vision of a Muslim woman wearing a hooded veil and a Detroit Lions sweatshirt and sweatpants.

Most striking was the overpowering smell. The air was absolutely fetid and attacked the nose with relentless aggression. Redolent with the scents of sixty people living under crowded conditions, combined with the remains of countless meals prepared in the kitchen just behind the staircase and a faulty toilet two floors above, it was not difficult for one's mind to be transported to a different time and place—such as a holding room at Ellis Island filled with immigrants who had just come off the steerage boats without bathing for a week or more.

The Ellis Island doctors, of course, lived in a period when one was hardly shy about making the obvious, if not crude, observation, "You stink!" They lived in an era that was closer to a time when many ascribed the spread of epidemic disease to miasmas—the smells and gases that emanated from rotting garbage, sewage, and even ill people.[10] Consequently, when confronted with the overpowering odor of so many unwashed bodies, those physicians often worried that such exposure might prove injurious to themselves or others.[11]

I crinkled my nose and slowed my breathing pattern as if such preemptive moves might protect me against invisible illness. Catching myself in my mind's eye, I tried to mask my revulsion with the equanimity of the doctor's visage, but I know a few, if not all, of the immigrants knew exactly what was going on in my head, so clearly were my thoughts being telegraphed. The sour smells, the broken toilet, and the anxiety and sadness that pervaded the crowded shelter that day served as a powerful reminder of how vastly different the lives of immigrants were (and are) from those of the American doctors assigned to their care.

One ritual that Lynne and I agreed upon was that we would have lunch with the residents each week before addressing their medical problems, to help all of us begin to get to know one another. Despite the unpleasant conditions of the dining area and the unappetizing fare, which consisted of surplus meat products, rice and beans, flat sodas, and a variety of other donated items, the meals were always prepared by the immigrants with joy and gusto.

After lunch, the real work began in a room upstairs that served as a clinic, office, and classroom for the immigrants. Along one wall was a giant glass-enclosed bookcase, each door padlocked, with many shelves of medications that were donated by well-intentioned pharmaceutical representatives. The bookcases presented a cornucopia of drugs ranging from antibiotics to powerful tranquilizers, many of them long past their expiration dates. Lisa, one of the social workers showing me around, noticed me staring with grave concern at the imprisoned and potentially unsafe stash. She reassured me: "Don't worry about those old medicines. We haven't been able to find the key to the locks for several months now." I made a mental note to gather together some essential medical staples for the Freedom House clinic before my next visit.

Lisa then displayed some of her teaching materials that she prepared for the newcomers' "basic hygiene" class. They included multilingual instruction booklets in Arabic, Russian, Spanish, French, Chinese, and Hindi, and a large doll with huge teeth that she used to help teach the immigrants how to brush and floss their teeth. While this is hardly a requisite course for all the refugees who come to Freedom House, it is important to note how many of them come from backgrounds where daily habits of personal hygiene can be markedly different from ours.

Lisa's hygiene class reminded me of a trip I had taken just a few weeks earlier to a dusty library in New York where I studied some yellowed and brittle copies of a newspaper entitled *School Health News*. This publication was distributed to New York City teachers during the peak of the first great wave of immigration to the United States in the early 1900s. Its purpose was to help them recognize and prevent illnesses among their pupils, and teach students (and, by extension, their foreign parents) about modern approaches to personal hygiene and health. One story described the work of an enterprising young nurse named Mrs. Stelljes.

She was assigned to P.S. 102, which was then situated in an Italian immigrant neighborhood in Manhattan. Armed with a wooden model of teeth built by her husband and a set of toothbrushes of varying size "for the different members of a family from the father down to the pre-school aged child," she visited the homes of her students to demonstrate how the toothbrush should be used and, more broadly, to preach on the "gospel" of hygiene.[12]

Today, of course, few Americans give much thought to the once major health problem of rotting teeth and its awful sequela: cavities, abscesses, nerve pain, and eating difficulties. Thanks to an enthusiastic cadre of dentists, dental hygienists, fluoridated water, the toothpaste industry, and modern aesthetic sensibilities surrounding our smile, it is easy to forget what a significant health problem this remains among the world's poorest citizens. "Not a bad place to start a course on health for our new residents, don't you think?" asked Lisa.

During my first several visits to Freedom House, there were no medical emergencies to speak of and I spent most of these afternoons simply talking to many of the residents.[13] Among my first "patients" were a trio of brothers who were born in Ethiopia, Musa, eighteen, Abraham, sixteen, and Tadelle, twelve. As a result of war and famine in the late 1980s, the boys, an older sister, and their mother fled to Windsor, Canada, by way of Saudi Arabia, the United Kingdom, and the United States. The boys have not seen their father since they were toddlers, and he is presumed to be dead.

During the late 1990s immigrant social services were far more expansive and easier to access in Canada than in the United States. As a result, Canada had become a destination for today's immigrants, as desirable as the United States once was only a century before. For six years, this refugee family lived in Windsor on a temporary visa. Their mother earned a living as a cook and a seamstress, and the boys went to school. Each spring the family received a letter from the Canadian immigration authorities requesting them to renew their visas. But seven months before we met, in May 1997, the Canadian officials asked the family to leave the country entirely and to begin the formal process of applying for permanent citizenship, as mandated by Canadian law. Because their transatlantic flight landed at Detroit Metropolitan Airport and the immigration authorities in Windsor ordered them to return to the last country they physically stepped foot in before arriving in Canada, the family wound up at Freedom House.

Musa, Abraham, and Tadelle, although Muslim, attended a Catholic parochial school connected to St. Anne's. Despite the confusing mélange of cultures, the boys mastered their circumstances with aplomb. In order to avoid the stigma of being "illegal aliens" they simply told their classmates they were "from Canada." Like so many young immigrants before them, these Ethiopian boys flowed from one persona and culture to the next, depending on what the immediate situation demanded, be it speaking with their mother, who knows little English and relies primarily on Arabic; their schoolmates, who are predominately Latino and African-American; their fellow residents at Freedom House, or visitors. They were citizens of the world who understood, better than most adults, that national boundaries are far more arbitrary and artificial than we care to admit.

The middle brother, Abraham, was an especially articulate and thoughtful young man. One afternoon, after a lunch of rice, fried eggs, and some type of greasy, leathery meat that defied his humorous attempts at identification, we went next door to the church's social hall to talk. The heat was out in Freedom House that day, so many of the residents were already eating in the slightly warmer social hall, which was filled with the noise of hammering as a group of young congregants built a theatrical set for their annual pageant. That year's show was entitled "Jesus in da' 'Hood." From the back of the hall, Abraham studiously observed a pack of teenagers painting a neon blue backdrop portraying a highly idealized skyline of Detroit with a giant Jesus Christ peering from behind a brightly lit Ambassador Bridge.

Huddled over lukewarm tea and with smoky vapor emerging from his mouth each time he exhaled, Abraham described his experiences at Freedom House and, more broadly, as a refugee moving from country to country without ever finding a permanent home:

> It's like being on one long monotonous train ride. Instead of a real train trip, this one has no destination. Only you don't know that at first. In fact, it took me a pretty long time before I realized that instead of being on a trip that went from point A to point B, I was really on a circular track that keeps going around and around. You see, the train stops at several points on the track. Newcomers get on and off. Like those four over there.

Abraham pointed to a young couple with two small children who had just arrived from Rwanda, and, while worn out and tired from their journey, they were clearly excited to be at Freedom House. He looked at the Rwandan family with equal parts compassion and sadness before continuing.

> But while you may be very excited to arrive—especially at the first few stops—soon enough, you realize that the path you are on is an endless circle. You never know when someone will get off and appear at your doorstep or if the conductor will tell them to get back on the train. Sometimes the train doors open and you're at a place like Freedom House or somewhere in Canada and you say, "This is it! I'm free! I can finally begin living my life!" But soon you have to get back on the train. By the third or fourth time around, you finally get the picture—at least I did.

There was no bitterness or rancor in Abraham's voice, simply wisdom that belied his young face. Indeed, he had brilliantly described the immigration experience as it currently unfolds for a multitude of people without papers or legal standing to make the migration process a bit easier. These refugees, especially those with little chance of being granted political asylum (a very difficult achievement even under the most extenuating circumstances of physical horror and danger), represent some of the saddest immigration stories today.

Shortly after this conversation with Abraham, his little brother, Tadelle, who wore baggy jeans three sizes too big for him and other accoutrements of the hip-hop generation, entered the room. Tadelle approached me suspiciously and asked if I was a lawyer. "No," I replied. "Are you an INS inspector?" Again I responded negatively and added that I was a doctor. Somewhat puzzled, Tadelle retorted, "They boot you out too?" We all laughed loudly at his wisecrack even as I explained I was a U.S. citizen merely visiting Freedom House. Nevertheless, Tadelle's observations of the refugee's world were almost as apt as his older brother's.

One Friday afternoon in late February, Lynne excitedly announced, "We just received twelve new residents from Rwanda and the Congo who I would like you to examine, but most of all I want you to see Yves. You've got to meet this young man because his story is so incredible."

Lynne ushered me into the residents' common room. Beyond the French doors were three threadbare and dusty sofas, a dilapidated recliner chair, and, dominating the room both in its bulk and the noise that came from it, a Zenith television. Judging from its style and the ornate "deluxe wooden cabinet" that surrounded the picture tube, the set was probably manufactured around 1960.

Yves was wearing an outfit donated to the shelter: an oversized, tattered Purdue University T-shirt and a pair of jeans that stopped several inches before his legs did. But it was only his wardrobe that lacked charm or style. There was a joy, a glow really, to Yves that was almost magnetic in its attraction. Six foot two in height, thin and muscular, Yves was an arrestingly good looking nineteen-year-old with unblemished ebony skin, delicate features, and intense brown eyes that proved to be a superb window to his emotional state over the next several months, ranging from unrestrained happiness during his first days at Freedom House, fear when recalling the horrors he left behind, boredom and dismay over the lengthy legal process to get a visa, to adolescent defiance.

Unlike many of the other African refugees we were seeing at Freedom House, Yves was the son of a successful businessman based in a small town on the border between Rwanda and what is today the Democratic Republic of the Congo. Coffee, tea, you name the valued commodity, and Yves's father found a way to bring it to market while making sure that a tidy profit went into his pocket. The family enjoyed all of the benefits of their father's success. They lived in a beautiful home. They wore expensive clothing imported from Italy and France. Yves and his two younger brothers were educated in the finest schools. The family took frequent trips to Europe, and they were all fluent in French, Spanish, and English. Only three years before, Yves was in Spain ostensibly to study, but like many teenagers blessed with such bounty, his real ambition was to "meet as many girls as I could and to party." To better illustrate the past he was describing, Yves passed around three wrinkled and worn photographs that he always kept in his back pocket: the first was a formal portrait of his family; the second, an exterior view of his home; and the third, a snapshot of him sporting a beaming smile in the center of a group of beautiful young women. His only commentary, "I missed my family that year, but I did very, very well in Spain."

We now know, of course, about the atrocities then occurring in Rwanda and the neighboring nations of Africa. Beginning in the spring of 1994, about one million or more Tutsis were murdered by armies of Hutus. But because these two groups share a common language, live among each other, and often intermarry, dividing the population of

Rwanda into Tutsis and Hutus was not a simple matter.[14] Whether one classified the Tutsis and Hutus as social groups, castes, or classes, however, they perceived themselves as quite distinct from one another, and an intense hatred often separated them.[15] There are many shocking aspects to the rampage of genocide that resulted from these perceived differences, to be sure, but one telling problem in our own country was just how indifferent many Americans were to these events as the news of the brutalities unfolded in real time.[16] For many, the Rwandan killing fields were merely headlines in the newspaper to be skimmed over as we sipped cups of freshly ground coffee each morning.[17]

Another Freedom House resident was a tall, beautiful, and extremely frightened twenty-four-year-old woman named Diannea. During the killing spree of 1994 the Hutus descended upon her tiny Tutsi village, armed with machetes and brawn, killing everything that moved and burning down as much of the village as possible.

Diannea was first raped by three soldiers and then hit repeatedly across the head, legs, and back. She passed out onto a pile of bodies. Leaving her for dead, the Hutus proceeded to other murderous tasks. Diannea regained consciousness within a few hours. In a most perverse version of the childhood game of possum, Diannea remained there, under several corpses, including her parents, "playing dead" until the Hutus left to attack another village. After an eighteen-month-long journey of exile and emigration out of Africa, to Spain and Italy, she finally reached the United States in late 1997. When we met, she was in the grip of a debilitating bout of what psychiatrists have named posttraumatic stress disorder. So easily shaken was she that the mere sound of a spoon dropped from the table and clattering onto the floor would drive her to tears. Tragically, Diannea's experiences were quite representative of the horrors going on in that part of the world at the time.

Around the time of Diannea's ordeal, in May 1994, Yves's father was brutally executed and the family home was burned to the ground. Yves heard about this while still in Spain, although he was uncertain whether the Hutu warriors or Congolese rebels perpetrated these murderous crimes. Along with this news, Yves was assured that his two younger brothers and mother had escaped and were in hiding. Several weeks after his arrival at Freedom House, however, Yves received word that they, too, were dead.

Yves left Spain for Portugal that fall with about $2,000 in cash and traveler's checks that was supposed to pay his tuition, room, and board.

In his hasty flight from Madrid, he lost his papers. Yves quickly realized that under the circumstances returning home to find his remaining family members or reapply for a passport was not a wise idea. Instead, he decided that his best chance for long-term survival was to travel to the United States. In order to earn the money he would need to make such an expensive journey, he began a three-year stint as a waiter and busboy in one of Lisbon's large hotels.

While in Lisbon, Yves "hooked up" with the immigration underground, a group of nefarious businessmen who sold everything a refugee might require to make a permanent trip to America: clothes, luggage, English lessons, plane tickets, and, most important, passports. One document merchant made Yves a particularly attractive and "foolproof" offer. For $5,000, this dealer would book Yves a coach ticket from Lisbon to John F. Kennedy Airport in New York. The travel package included the "rental" of a Portuguese passport that was professionally doctored to feature Yves's photo on the identification page. Once the two men made it through customs at JFK, Yves was required to hand back the forged passport to the dealer, who then promptly boarded a return flight back to Lisbon to begin the process anew with another aspiring immigrant.[18]

In fact, the "rental" of travel documents is hardly a rare event. For those with means but without a bona fide passport, it is a popular way to arrange a quick exit out of one country to another. This arrangement, however, not only left Yves in a financially precarious situation; it also deposited him in the middle of a busy international airport, literally feet away from several U.S. Customs and immigration officers, without a shred of identification or legitimate legal status to be there.

Yves took a dramatic pause in his narration, although everyone listening was clearly on the edge of his or her seat wondering what happened next. He confidently smiled, scanned the faces of his audience, and finally resumed with the observation: "I knew I was in trouble, but it was a long trip. I walked through the airport and soon I saw a giant, what do they call it, food court? There was a wonderful pizza place there. So I went over, sat down, and ordered a large one, with everything. And a beer. It was delicious."

Charming might well have been Yves's middle name. At the pizzeria, he sidled up next to two young women who were returning to New York from a year of studying abroad. After thirty minutes of pizza, beer, and a complete recounting of his life story, the young women decided to help him. "Do you know anyone in the United States?" they asked. "Do you have anywhere to go?" Yves recalled the document dealer saying that Canada was a much more hospitable destination for refugees than the United States, but the fee for a trip to Toronto was $6,500 rather than the $5,000 Yves could barely afford. He also remembered the document dealer mentioning that some immigrants went to Detroit as a pathway to Canada. And so Yves told his newfound friends that he would like to go to Detroit.

The young women pooled together a few hundred dollars and instructed Yves how to get into Manhattan and, specifically, to the Port Authority Bus Terminal. Once there, he purchased a ticket and boarded a bus for Detroit. There was just one problem Yves did not consider: if he wanted to enter Canada via Detroit he would need a passport or some official form of identification. It was not until two days later, when the Greyhound bus wheeled into the downtown Detroit bus station and he could see through the window the American and Canadian flags waving from the roof of the U.S. Customs Building that he realized the gravity of his tactical error.

But Yves was nothing if not a successful immigrant. The annals of the American immigration experience are replete with such souls who make the best of every situation and rely upon their wits, personalities, and charm to wriggle out of tight situations that would bring most of us to our knees. Yves explained, sitting in the living room of Freedom House, that he simply did not have time to wallow in dejection or self-pity. He wandered the streets of Detroit for three days, took his meals at a soup kitchen, and spent a few nights in a shelter for the homeless before heading to the west side of the city, where he could see the Ambassador Bridge. Once he got there, he looked longingly across the span, thinking if only he could get to Canada he might be safe and his long nightmare might finally end. That night, he slept outside in a small park near the bridge, a few blocks from Freedom House. It was bitter cold and Yves was quite hungry. The following morning he came across a local police precinct and decided to go inside. It turned out to be one of the most fortuitous decisions he would ever make on American soil.

Seated inside the battered, old precinct house was a forty-five-year-old African-American police sergeant who had a son about Yves's age. The cop looked up from his desk and asked Yves what he wanted. The tall, good-looking, but obviously distressed refugee explained his story of tragedy and flight. After locating the forms required when encountering illegal aliens, the police officer began asking the standard questions that typically led to a refugee being whisked off to a jail until a hearing was held to decide his ultimate fate. "What is your name?" "Where is your place of birth?" "What is your date of birth?" Mundane questions to be sure, but it was this last question that turned out to be Yves's "open sesame" to America.

"July 4, 1979," replied Yves. The policeman's pen and jaw dropped simultaneously and he replied: "Friend, this is your lucky day." He tore up the INS forms, put on his coat, and drove Yves to Freedom House, where Lynne Partington accepted him at once and agreed to help prepare his asylum case. This experience was less than forty-eight hours old the afternoon Yves recounted his story, and he was clearly euphoric over his good fortune.

As a cold, gray, and bleak February passed into an equally cold, gray, and bleak March, a blanket of depression covered the residents of Freedom House. Whether one called it "the winter blues," "seasonal affective disorder," or "an appreciation of reality," it was striking after my initial visits to be welcomed exclusively by the sad faces and spirit that now enveloped the shelter. Rwandans, Congolese, Ethiopians, Palestinians, Iraqis, Salvadorans, Guatemalans, Nicaraguans, and all the other refugees simply stared into space or at the constantly blaring television, ate mechanically, and were bored out of their minds. Few of the residents read or even had anything worth reading. Only two newly arrived families, one from Poland and the other from Russia, seemed to take the cold weather in stride and ventured outside for daily bundled walks in the neighborhood. For most of the residents, Freedom House had become a jail. The windows were shut tightly, the doors locked, and the air close and acrid. The days passed slowly as their worries grew exponentially.

The person most affected by this situation was Yves. Merely engaging him in a conversation more extensive than monosyllabic replies of "yes" or "no" was now an all but impossible task. Gone was the glow of success he exuded that first afternoon when recounting his flight from Africa and Europe, not to mention his adventures courtesy of the Detroit Police Department. In less than a month, Yves had transformed into a bitter and angry young man.

Yves grew steadily obsessed with and resentful of the "strict rules" imposed upon him at Freedom House. He began fighting with some of the other residents, and exhibited the outraged and petulant manner that adolescents all over the world master so easily. In his mind, Lynne Partington had transmogrified from "my favorite American lady" into "my most hated enemy." Lynne was quite used to such transference of feelings. She had, after all, worked with immigrants and refugees for many years. But the stress on her face whenever she discussed Yves's case was difficult to hide.

The change in Yves's behavior, of course, was related directly to his realization that he was going to be in Freedom House for a long time before any resolution was reached. By this point, he had spent many long hours talking with the other immigrants and learning about their plights. He was now beginning to understand the circularity and tedium of the never-ending "train ride" that refugees like Abraham had long since accepted as the baseline of their existence. While the shelter was certainly not as horrible as he described, the shabby living conditions, the strict rules governing his every act, the communal meals, and the intense boredom that now characterized the place for him were difficult to accept.

Yves's rebellion seemed to intensify on an hourly basis. In late March he announced that he had taken a job as a stock boy in a tiny market owned by a Mexican-American man a few blocks from the shelter. The shop owner, who himself had immigrated to the United States only ten years earlier, saw no moral or legal problems in his employment practices, and often tried to recruit Freedom House residents and illegal aliens to work in his bodega. Although Lynne and her staff members repeatedly warned the residents against even thinking about taking such positions, Yves was seduced by the seemingly princely sum of $2 an hour and free Cokes. When Lynne discovered that Yves and two other teenaged boys, one from Lebanon and the other from Nicaragua, were working at the bodega, she told them in no uncertain terms to quit immediately. Her concern stemmed from the fact that even such a low-level job violated their refugee status with the INS.

Despite Lynne's admonitions, Yves continued to steal away a few hours a day to work at the bodega for almost a month. Things became even more problematic when Lynne discovered that the shop owner paid his help not with cash, but by check. Yves had, by now, mastered a common practice of the American urban poor who do not have bank accounts: going to a check-cashing center where a sour, taciturn banker, protected by a double pane of safety glass, cashed any check presented, provided the recipient turned over a healthy percentage as his fee. All of these financial transactions left a splendid paper trail of immigration violations that the Freedom House staffers worried might haunt Yves when he finally did get an asylum hearing before the INS magistrate. But the concrete (some might call it hardheaded) reasoning of a teenager, particularly one who had escaped the violence and torture Yves did, combined with the normal risk-taking behavior that characterizes adolescence, rendered their pleas unconvincing. And because he was legally considered an adult, there was pitifully little they could do to stop him from pursuing these activities. Fortunately for Yves, the bodega owner was equally unscrupulous in actually paying his help. After two skipped pay periods, Yves finally quit on his own.

It was around this time that news of the murders of his mother and two younger brothers finally reached Yves. Heartbroken and devastated, Yves refused to eat, rarely left the tiny bedroom he shared with three other boys, and spent most of his days crying. The rest of us who all fervently wanted to help him had absolutely no idea of how to go about it. What do you say to a young man whose entire family has been slaughtered? What possible act of kindness or words of advice could ever assuage the horror of such an unimaginable atrocity? The recent arrival of several families from Rwanda to Freedom House was a small blessing in Yves's grieving process. At least now he had people near him who could understand his ordeal completely.

Only a few weeks after Yves learned about the death of the rest of his family and the arrival of the Rwandan families, I received an urgent phone call from one of the Freedom House workers, an unflappable, dedicated young woman who was working on her master's degree in social work. She had been at Freedom House for three years and, like the other staff members, had a wealth of experience managing situations that veered perilously between bad and worse. But on this morning her voice almost vibrated with panic as she explained that there was a serious "outbreak of something" in the house.

"Outbreak? Outbreak of what?" I asked nervously. "What do you mean?" The staff worker then went on to explain how the night before, one of the Rwandan children, Ollie, developed a severe case of diarrhea that simply would not abate. To make matters worse, by morning, Ollie's little brother, Otto, a teenaged boy named Charles, and Yves were experiencing the same problem. I asked whether or not the boys were all sleeping in the same room, and she replied affirmatively. Apparently, they were rewarded that night with a large pizza along with some other takeout goodies because they did such a great job cleaning up the bathrooms earlier that day.

At this point she asked if I thought there was some kind of medical connection. "I don't know," I replied. But even though I answered noncommittally, I immediately thought about the plethora of cholera cases then being discovered in the Rwandan refugee camps. "When was the most recent arrival of a Rwandan from one of the camps to Freedom House?" I asked. Unfortunately, she gave me the answer I most dreaded: "Only a few days ago."

In retrospect, I am not entirely sure I believed that cholera had struck Freedom House, but the period between possibly contracting the infection in an African refugee camp and the appearance of the diarrhea made for a compelling clinical scenario. Indeed, the incubation period for cholera can be within hours to about five days after exposure. I ended the telephone conversation by telling her to try to get the children to drink as much as possible and that I'd be there in an hour. Before I left Ann Arbor, I called one of my hospital's infectious disease specialists. He agreed that the situation needed to be investigated but seriously doubted my preliminary diagnosis. "Cholera in Detroit?" the infectious disease expert exclaimed. "That's one for the medical journals."


Cholera is a disease I was well acquainted with as a historian but one I had never seen in my medical practice. Many times over the years when my pager beeped me to the hospital's emergency room, it was a call from a physician entertaining a diagnosis of a "historical" disease that with the advances of medicine has been all but conquered in the United States today. Cholera, yellow fever, diphtheria, plague, typhus, polio—these were the infectious killers that my professional forebears dreaded and encountered with chilling regularity. Today, however, my medical students (and many of my colleagues in practice) can barely pronounce or spell their antiquated names, let alone recognize a case that might walk into their clinics. Thus far, not a single one of these diagnostic exercises has resulted in the positive identification of a classic scourge, yet my colleagues and I always have a good time considering them.

But cholera was high on my list of differential diagnoses as I drove into Detroit for more than quaint historical reasons. Most important were the reams of epidemiological reports between 1994 and 1998 that described numerous outbreaks of cholera in the Rwandan refugee camps and along other points of the African emigration path.[19] In fact, cholera appears with great regularity in the world today, particularly after the destruction of water lines and sewage facilities, whether by natural disasters or human means (most typically war). A 1995 World Health Organization report identified it as one of the world's "top ten" infectious killers, along with typhoid, dysentery, tuberculosis, malaria, hepatitis B, HIV/AIDS, measles, tetanus, pertussis, and intestinal parasites.[20]

Cholera has circled the globe many times. From the days of the ancient Greeks until the final years of the nineteenth century, it was one of the most feared (and disgusting) killers known. At least seven times in modern history, cholera swept throughout the world, often beginning in the Indian subcontinent and Middle East, moving westward through Asia and Russia, on to Europe and, in 1832, 1849, and 1866, across the Atlantic Ocean. In the New World, it usually struck first in New York City, the major port of the United States, before fanning out along the eastern seaboard, the Midwest, and beyond. This is precisely the path the scourge took in 1832, when Father Gabriel Richard, tending to his parish at St. Anne's in Detroit, was silenced forever.[21]

*Cholera: "The Kind of 'Assisted Emigrant' We Can Not Afford to Admit"*

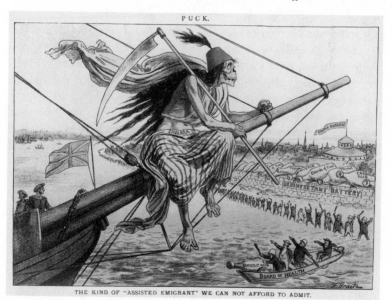

THE KIND OF "ASSISTED EMIGRANT" WE CAN NOT AFFORD TO ADMIT.

The American view of cholera as a completely foreign disease was per-haps best personified in a cartoon published in an 1883 issue of the humor magazine *Puck*.[22] This lavish illustration depicts a cholera-ridden skeleton wearing a Turkish fez and exotic pantaloons confidently astride the mast of a ship coming into New York harbor. Prepared to meet the cholera are armed, uniformed sanitary police stationed along Manhat-tan's "Disinfectant Battery" with a magazine of cannons labeled "chloride of lime," "sulphur," and "carbolic acid," aimed directly at the disease-ridden ship. The cartoon's caption further clarifies this hardly subtle image: "The Kind of 'Assisted Emigrant' We Can Not Afford to Admit."

All of these worldwide pandemics and their resultant panic were caused by the *Vibrio cholerae*, a tiny, comma-shaped bacterium with an even tinier whiplike tail that allows it to swim about in the water. When the germ is present in drinking water or on the surface of food washed with contaminated water, even the most robust person can be knocked down and out within a matter of hours.

In the late 1840s an assertive British physician named John Snow challenged the long-standing medical opinion that foul-smelling vapors emanating from mounds of rotting garbage and human and animal waste, a common feature of most urban centers of this era, caused cholera. Snow's fascination with the disease began when he encountered it professionally in the seaport town of Sunderland near Newcastle in 1831. Twenty-three years later, he tracked down the source of London's great cholera epidemic of 1854 by meticulously surveying every case and their contacts even to the point of verifying their water source by check-ing each home's water bills. What the doctor discovered was that the Londoners who drew water from the Southwark and Vauxhall Water Company, which came from the fecal-contaminated Thames River, were infected nine times more than those in areas supplied by the Lambeth Company, whose water originated from an upstream (and less contami-nated) source.[23]

Even more dramatic was Snow's study of cholera's effect on his neigh-borhood in the Soho parish of London. After carefully charting the five hundred cholera cases in his district, Dr. Snow noted that most of the cholera victims consumed water from a well located in Broad Street. Unfortunately for those who frequented the hand pump–operated well, it was contaminated with sewage from a nearby house where cholera had already visited. Snow convinced the parish councilors to remove the well's pump handle, thus making it inoperable. Soon after, the cholera

rate in Soho fell dramatically. Snow's conclusion was that a specific living, waterborne "poison" capable of self-reproduction was in the excreta
and vomitus of the cholera patients who, in turn, tainted the water
supply. The young doctor's solution was simple but effective: washing
hands thoroughly, decontaminating soiled linens, and boiling drinking
water.[24] Alas, only three years after publishing his seminal paper on the
cause of cholera, the forty-five-year-old physician dropped dead from a
cerebral hemorrhage. It would take almost thirty years and a series of
scientific discoveries into the world of microbes and human disease
before Dr. Snow's brilliant detective work was proven definitively.

That moment came during the summer of 1883 when cholera struck
Calcutta and Bombay before traveling westward through Egypt. By
June, the scourge struck Dumyat along the Nile Delta, midway between
Port Said and Alexandria. The epidemic's timing was propitious for the
microbe, if not human beings, because it arrived exactly when an annual
festival was being held in the town which attracted most of its 30,000
inhabitants and an additional 15,000 visitors.

Under the best of circumstances, Dumyat was not exactly a sanitary
town. One observer in 1883 noted that "the air [was] odorous with nau-
seating and miasmatic vapors." Another complained that "the streets
were defiled with fecal filth," and even more disturbing, "Arab children
take off their scanty clothing, enter the puddles in the streets, play,
bathe, and roll in them, and come out covered from head to foot in a
coating of mud and mire." Not surprisingly, within a week of cholera's
arrival to the town, more than a hundred Egyptians were dying each day.
During the early days of the epidemic some 25,000 townsmen and visitors fled with their lives to other parts of Egypt. By the week's close, a
cordon of armed soldiers closed off the town's boundaries to block the
passage of all those trying to leave and, tragically, the delivery of goods,
food, and medicine into Dumyat. As with almost every quarantine
erected in human history, the infection still managed to escape the
hastily drawn boundaries, traveling first to Cairo, Alexandria, and Port
Said, and from there, to the ports of Marseilles, Toulon, Genoa, and
Naples, where it claimed an additional 50,000 lives.[25]

In early August a team of German bacteriologists led by Robert Koch
was dispatched to Alexandria. Once there, Koch organized a careful
series of autopsies on the cholera victims. He had more than enough
cadavers to choose from, and he became especially fascinated by the victims' ravaged guts. After a thorough microscopic analysis of the dead

Egyptians' gastrointestinal tracts, Dr. Koch noted that they were riddled with a comma-shaped bacterium. A few days later a special team of investigators who worked in Louis Pasteur's laboratory in Paris joined the Koch team.

One of the French bacteriologists, Louis Thuillier, was stricken by cholera and succumbed to the microbe on September 19. Appropriately, Koch was at the young investigator's deathbed and served as a pallbearer at Thuillier's funeral the following morning. But that very afternoon Dr. Koch was back at his makeshift laboratory, where he created a variety of methods to artificially grow the comma-shaped bacteria, *Vibrio cholerae*, in culture and prove that they were the cause of widespread diarrheal misery. The following year, during a repeat epidemic in Toulon, Koch replicated his findings, and on July 26, 1884, he formally announced them to the world.

Up until relatively recently, it was assumed that the vibrio lodged in the gut of a victim, and steadily shredded and sloughed the intestinal lining, rendering the human gut useless and resulting in massive, painful, dehydrating diarrhea. East European Jews apparently understood this etiological theory all too well, because a common curse in their Yiddish lexicon was the euphonious *Zol a cholerye dir choppen; a brannt dir in di kishkes a bruch dir indigedaynm,* or roughly translated: "May you be seized by the cholera and there should be by you a burning in the intestines and a breaking of the guts."[26] A picturesque phrase, to be sure, though hardly lyrical enough to be included in the candy-coated version of *shtetl* life that was widely popularized in the Broadway musical version of Sholom Aleichem's "Tevye the Dairyman" stories, *Fiddler on the Roof.*[27]

Interestingly, subsequent investigations disproved this hypothesis. In the late 1950s physicians developed an instrument called the endoscope, which allowed them to snake a tube into a patient's gastrointestinal tract for a closer look and the possible diagnosis of disease. Enchanted by this technological advance, in 1960 a curious gastroenterologist named Eugene Gangarosa and a few of his colleagues used the newly developed endoscope on cholera patients shipped in from South America to the Walter Reed Hospital in Washington, D.C. The purpose of their research was to actually observe the intestinal walls of these cholera patients. What they found out was that no such bloody warfare was occurring at all.[28]

Instead, as it was later discovered, the microbe employs a far craftier means of destruction. *Vibrio cholerae* toxin is composed of two subunits prosaically named enterotoxin subunit A and, you guessed it, enterotoxin subunit B. It is subunit B that allows the organism to irreversibly bind to specific receptors on cells that line the small intestine. Once attached, the organism multiplies with the wanton abandon expected of bacteria and injects subunit A, a powerful poison, into the small intestine's epithelial cells, one layer below. The toxin activates an enzyme in the cells called adenylate cyclase, which then turns on another powerful catalyst called $3'$ $5'$-cyclic adenosine monophosphate. The result of these chemical reactions is a virtual flood of the critical electrolytes sodium and potassium into the bowel, followed by an actual flood of the body's water stores—the principal ingredient of all living things. Ironically, the cholera germ's talent for wreaking pathological havoc is a borrowed trait. All of the genes that code for the vibrio's ability to create the toxin responsible for inducing this massive fluid loss originate from a bacteriophage—a virus that prefers bacteria to humans—that infected and incorporated itself into the cholera's genome long, long ago.[29]

Regardless of origin, this toxin unleashes a veritable Niagara of foul-smelling, mucous-flecked, watery diarrhea. So profound is this unlofty surge that nineteenth-century physicians who did not yet have access to modern means of intravenous fluid replacement simply placed their patients on a "cholera bed," a canvas cot with a hole cut in its center and a large bucket directly below it. The clear expectation of these doctors was that the patient would soon die of dehydration. It was, as historian Richard Evans describes, "a vulgar and demeaning disease. Its reputation as a disease of the poor only strengthened its repulsiveness."[30]

How repulsive? Let's review, for a moment, the actual experience of cholera. Like many illnesses, it begins simply with the vague sense of not feeling well. Soon after this intuition of illness, maybe three to six hours later, come violent waves of diarrhea and, often, vomiting. So forceful are the choleraic propulsions from both ends of the gut that the victim experiences intense, painful spasms of the abdominal muscles that even a casual observer looking at a cholera patient's belly can see. It's almost as if the squirming thew and sinew have taken on a life of their own.

In a matter of hours, the relentless diarrhea gives way to dehydration and shock. Internally, the kidneys shut down their operations because the body's lack of water directly translates into a lack of blood flow.

Crudely put, without blood to filter, the kidneys have no urine to make. The circulation system becomes flaccid and sluggish. In distant regions, the arteries collapse. With continued water loss, the blood itself can thicken, sludge, and even clot. Pulses weaken, and, ultimately, tissues and organs die.

Externally, the victim's face turns pinched and blue, the voice faint and high-pitched, the mouth and lips parched and cracked, and the eyes deeply sunken, giving off a surreal and ghostlike appearance. Without the life-giving intervention of intravenous (IV) fluids, the patient's vitality only wanes further as the diarrhea increases, accompanied by a clouded sense of reality, more spasms, seizures, and coma. Even today, in parts of the world where IV fluids are not readily available, 25 to 50 percent of all cholera patients die; when these lifesaving treatments are available, the mortality rate drops to 1 to 5 percent.

But the real problem, of course, is that cholera refuses to retire to the dusty pages of an old medical textbook. Since 1961 the world has witnessed the seventh great pandemic and the major culprit is the El Tor biotype of *Vibrio cholerae* that was first isolated that year in Sulawesi, Indonesia. Since then it has spread rapidly throughout Asia, Europe, and Africa before reaching South America in 1991, when more than 400,000 cases and 4,000 deaths were reported in 16 different Latin American countries. In late 1992 a new strain of *Vibrio cholerae* called 0139 Bengal was discovered, and more than 100,000 cases of cholera were reported in India and Bangladesh. This variant has since spread to Pakistan, Afghanistan, Nepal, and through much of Southeast Asia.

During 1994 a major epidemic of cholera occurred in a refugee camp in Goma, Democratic Republic of the Congo, and 80,000 cases and 23,800 deaths were reported in one month. Sadly, the story hardly ends there. Between 1997 and 1998 there was a twofold increase in cholera around the world, and the "hottest zone" of all was Africa. In 1998, 211,748 cases of cholera were reported in the Democratic Republic of the Congo, Rwanda, Kenya, Mozambique, Uganda, Tanzania, and other parts of Africa, accounting for 72 percent of the world's total cases. As the World Health Organization noted in late 2001, "the seventh pandemic is still ongoing and shows signs of increasing further rather than abating."[31]

A much broader public health concern stems from the fact that our planet's water supply is declining steadily. At present, we use more than half the world's accessible fresh water, and by 2025 we are likely to use

75 percent. Today, more than 1.5 billion people lack ready access to clean drinking water, and by 2025 that number may rise to 3.5 billion. Factor in the contamination of freshwater supplies, and matters only become more alarming. In developing nations, for example, more than 90 percent of wastewater is discharged without treatment of any kind directly into streams and rivers, and each year there are more than 250 million cases of water-related diseases worldwide, with 5 to 10 million cases resulting in death.[32] Therefore, it did not seem unreasonable that April morning to entertain the notion that if cholera was going to make an appearance in the United States, it was likely to have traveled by way of Congo, Rwanda, or one of the other disease-stricken regions of Africa.

When I finally pulled up in front of Freedom House, I was nervous. I had little in my doctor's bag save my stethoscope, a never-used bandage scissors (but no bandages), some tongue depressors, specimen cups, and a prescription pad. Two staff workers were waiting for me at the door. Before I even made it up the steps of the house's porch, they fretfully updated me about the four boys and their abrupt onset of diarrhea.

When I walked into the house, the same group of immigrants I saw only a week earlier greeted me. There were no smiles, no hellos, and despite the silence, a clear communication of fear. Mothers held their children close to them as if a maternal hug might protect their charges from contracting whatever had entered their home. Others simply averted their eyes, perhaps in the hope that avoiding a doctor might help them escape the mysterious disease.

The practice of medicine at Freedom House was far closer to that of the late nineteenth century than the late 1990s. There were neither X-rays nor laboratory tests to confirm or deny potential diagnoses. There were no prepared IV fluids, let alone the needles, tubing, and tape required to set up such a procedure. And while I spent the better part of my internship inserting IV needles into the tiny veins of infants and children, I had not "started a line" in about eight years. So even with the right equipment, my success in treating the patients I was about to greet was doubtful.

By the time I got to the second landing of the serpentine staircase, I was hit by the overpowering stench of several people stricken with diarrhea. The odor came in waves that were almost visible. And just as I did the first time I entered Freedom House, I temporarily held my breath as if merely inhaling the disgusting vapors into my lungs might cause me harm.

The four boys were lying on cots in the same tiny room. Buckets were placed near their beds, and some were filled with murky brown water. I first approached the youngest boys because they were at greatest risk of dehydrating due to their size. While they had dry chapped lips, their physical examinations were not compatible with any other signs of severe dehydration. The same could also be said for the eighteen-year-old young man with diarrhea.

My good friend Yves was the most obviously ill person in the room. Moaning and clutching his stomach, he appeared to be in great distress. But on further examination, even Yves did not appear to be dehydrated to the point that he needed to be transferred to a hospital immediately.

I asked one of the aides to get me some of the soda pop they had stored in the refrigerator. The surplus brands donated to Freedom House almost always came in syrupy-sweet varieties, like grape or strawberry. Pouring out four large cups and a smaller one for myself, I asked the four boys to begin taking small sips every few minutes and stayed to make sure they were able to hold the liquid down.

Without access to a microscope to look at the diarrheal stools the boys were producing, I had no objective evidence that the comma-shaped bacterium *Vibrio cholerae* was, in fact, the culprit. But this no longer mattered. Despite a clinical scenario that was not entirely consistent with the signs and symptoms of cholera, I had already formed a conclusion. The propensity for germs to travel, the fact that the other Rwandans had just arrived from refugee camps where there were reports of cholera outbreaks, and the many historical episodes swimming in my head all led to one answer: Yves and the boys must be suffering from cholera. Q.E.D.

I asked the residents curiously gawking at the doorway to stay away from the boys' bedroom and the nearby bathroom. Without announcing the ominous diagnosis I was entertaining in my mind, I was completely nonplussed as to how to proceed. Initially, I leaped to the idea of ordering a strict quarantine of the house, even though I knew that it was not likely to do much good. As the great pathologist William Henry Welch observed in 1893: "the achievements of quarantine in keeping out cholera have been relative to its vexations, hardships, cruelties, and interference with commerce so small that many distinguished sanitarians would discard it altogether."[33] For an even briefer moment, I was tempted to call 911 to arrange for an ambulance to take the four boys to a local hospital for intravenous fluids and treatment more definitive than the slow slurping of flat grape soda I was offering them. There is, after all, a purposeful excitement to the arrival of an ambulance, the attention-grabbing scream of a siren, the rushing entry of paramedics, the opening and slamming of doors, the clattering of collapsible gurneys, and the yelling—always the yelling—of emergency technicians barking orders to one another and those around them. But something held me back from dialing.

Instead, I asked each boy to give me a sample of his stools in the little plastic cups I had in the bottom of my doctor's bag and instructed one of the aides to make sure the boys continued to slowly drink as much as they could hold. I drove the specimens myself to a local hospital in order to get a better sense of what exactly was causing the outbreak of diarrhea.

The hospital was only about a mile away, and I went directly into the emergency room, where I introduced myself and explained what I was after. Amid a gaggle of shockingly young interns and residents, bedecked in green scrub suits and with stethoscopes rakishly wrapped around their necks like magical amulets, the charge nurse asked me to wait in the "visitor's area" while one of the physicians analyzed the specimens under the ER's microscope. Although I complied, I instantly hated this woman, unknown to me before and since this brief encounter, for so quickly relegating me to the lowly status of "visitor." Like countless "civilians" forced to sit out in a doctor's waiting room, I picked up a months-old magazine to waste some time and calm my nerves. What seemed like hours later, a senior resident came out to the waiting room to speak to me. He looked about eighteen years old, even though he was at least thirty, and in what I perceived to be a dismissive tone, asked, "Doctor, who said these guys have cholera?"

"Well," I stammered, knowing exactly where this dialogue was headed, "no one made a definitive diagnosis, per se, it's just that given the constellation of symptoms, and that some of the patients recently lived in a Rwandan refugee camp, it was a concern. . . ." As I trailed off in volume and conviction, the younger doctor smiled in a way I know I have smiled at physicians who referred a patient to me with a grossly incorrect diagnosis. He somewhat sarcastically uttered the word "rota" as he turned on his heels and walked away back into the treatment area.

By "rota," he meant rotavirus—one of the most common causes of diarrhea in the world. No minor footnote to a medical textbook, rotavirus is responsible for more than 140 million episodes of diarrhea per year and 1 million deaths worldwide. In the United States alone, there are more than 3.5 million cases annually, and 50,000 of these are severe enough to warrant hospitalization. Each winter and spring almost every American pediatrician sees dozens, if not hundreds, of cases— miserable little kids with "the runs" and exhausted parents searching for an end to the foul-smelling diarrheal river they've been desperately trying to dam. And while our country is blessed with superb hospitals and medical care, specifically the administration of intravenous fluids, this gastrointestinal virus continues to kill about 100 American children a year.[34]

But the two-syllable diagnosis "rota" demonstrated far more than the fact that my initial call of cholera was incorrect. The word screamed— even if only I could hear the shouting—"You fool, you made the assumption that these immigrants imported cholera when they were suffering from a form of diarrhea that is as American, if markedly less palatable, as apple pie."

Back when I was in medical school, I knew a professor who was particularly fond of a peculiar axiom: "When you hear the sound of hoofbeats, it is probably horses rather than zebras." Like many a native-born American treating foreign patients, I chose to track down a zebra rather than a local horse. I had envisioned the very real epidemics of cholera that had been reported in Africa and South America over the past few years. From my viewpoint, I was convinced—or I convinced myself— that the threat of imported infection was imminent. And this was an excellent lesson to experience firsthand. It was only at Freedom House that I began to appreciate how difficult it is to protect the public's health against the ingress of so-called foreign germs without overlooking the health threats that often exist in our own backyards. Although they could have easily done so, not a single *Vibrio cholerae* microbe traveled across the ocean. At least, not *this* time. These immigrants contracted their malady in my hometown, Detroit.

# EPILOGUE
## "Public Health Is Purchasable"

Disease is largely a removable evil. It continues to afflict humanity, not only because of incomplete knowledge of its causes and lack of adequate individual and public hygiene, but also because it is extensively fostered by harsh economic and industrial conditions and by wretched housing in congested communities. These conditions and consequently the diseases which spring from them can be removed by better social organization. No duty of society, acting through its governmental agencies, is paramount to this obligation to attack the removable causes of disease.... Public health is purchasable.

—HERMANN M. BIGGS, M.D., 1911[1]

Though not exactly a household name, in his day Hermann M. Biggs wielded enormous power and influence both in the United States and abroad. Throughout his distinguished career as general medical officer of the New York City Health Department and, subsequently, the commissioner of health of the state of New York, Dr. Biggs developed creative and effective policies that found reasonable compromises between protecting the public health and respecting the needs of the ill.

Biggs's entire career was framed by the new and exciting discoveries being made about microbes, beginning with Robert Koch's stunning 1882 announcement on the cause of tuberculosis. An event that occurred during Biggs's student days at Bellevue Medical College in New York City illustrates the cultural and intellectual wedge then being driven between old-fashioned medicine and the scientific revolution that continues to the present day.

One of Biggs's medical school professors was Dr. William Henry Welch, then a brilliant young pathologist eager to dedicate his academic pursuits to the science of bacteriology. On a spring afternoon Welch demonstrated Koch's discovery of the tubercle bacillus to his laboratory class, of which Biggs was a promising member. So inspired by this pedagogic moment, Biggs and a few of his classmates ran to the senior professor at Bellevue, the grand old man of New York medicine, Alfred L. Loomis, to tell him about it. A few days later the doubting Professor Loomis ascended the lecture platform of the Bellevue Hospital amphitheater, looked merrily about the vast room, and posited authoritatively:

"People say there are bacteria in the air, but I cannot see them." The young men in the audience less imbued with germ theory than Hermann Biggs laughed uproariously at Loomis's witty denunciation. But when Biggs recounted the story to Dr. Welch the pathologist noted presciently: "That's too bad. Loomis is such a nice man."[2] Dr. Welch understood that time had passed the senior physician by; older ideas of disease causation or prevention had been, or were about to be, superseded by new ones. Those who refused to accept these ideas would soon be relics.

Many years after their days at Bellevue, William Henry Welch was assigned the difficult task of delivering a eulogy at his former pupil's funeral. Welch noted that Biggs was "tenacious of principles in which he believed, patiently perseverant and fearless, without aggressiveness, constructive and clear in vision, with a sure sense of the immediately attainable."[3] These characteristics should be considered the quintessential job qualification for a public health official of any era. Dr. Biggs accomplished many remarkable scientific achievements during his career. His greatest contribution, by far, was his insistence that for every public health venture under his supervision the operative word was "public." Biggs knew that without generating a strong consensus among the multitudes that constitute a community, little could be accomplished in any attempt to rein in disease.

With the passage of a century, public health administration is markedly different, thanks to the relentless advances in technology and transportation. When Biggs was supervising the public health of America's largest metropolis in 1892, an epidemic raging among newly arrived immigrants in New York harbor primarily alarmed residents living no farther away than the northern reaches of Manhattan. But, then again, steamship travel from a European port to New York City took seven to ten days. Today, we are only beginning to appreciate that the health conditions in Africa or the former Soviet Union are intimately tied to those in Detroit or Los Angeles.

Pronouncements like Biggs's on the intimate, if not causal, relationship between economic or living conditions and epidemic diseases were made long before he put pen to paper and, of course, continue to be made in the present. Yet too little is being done by wealthier nations to ameliorate these conditions worldwide, even though they will ultimately affect the affluent as well as the poor. Not surprisingly, it was an immigrant, Abraham Cahan, who best characterized the American social response to the acute rise and fall of epidemic diseases. Cahan, a

Yiddish-speaking journalist who settled in New York City's Lower East Side, wrote the following passage during the cholera epidemic of 1892 while sitting in the city room of the *New York Arbeiter Zeitung*, a weekly socialist newspaper published by the Hebrew Trade Union. His words could have been jotted down today just as easily and, most likely, tomorrow:

> The American public's concern about unsanitary living conditions and related social problems of the downtrodden seem to get attention only when such epidemics threaten to creep into the palaces of the rich. Once a crisis passes over, the wealthy people's awareness of such problems becomes dormant and it is not until another extraordinary danger arises that fear and panic awaken their senses again.[4]

Pathogenic microbes do not discriminate, even if many are more likely to set up shop in the homes of the extremely poor and malnourished. Regardless of the contagious threat, from bioterrorist attacks of anthrax, mosquito-borne West Nile fever or malaria, waterborne cholera and *Salmonella* to the more ubiquitous AIDS and tuberculosis and the still somewhat exotic but always dramatic Ebola, the human race is simply too interconnected to rely on walls or borders as public health safeguards. The recent battle against severe acute respiratory syndrome (SARS) and its cause, a newly emerging strain of coronavirus, demonstrates how germs can spread across the global village brilliantly. Quarantines, cordons sanitaires, immigration depots, and long inspection lines all represent a past era's responses to the containment of contagion. Today, these antiquated approaches are no longer up to the job.

Around the world today, 10 million children die each year, and almost a third of these deaths are due to infectious diseases and maternal or perinatal conditions. Approximately 1.6 million of the childhood deaths could be wholly prevented with immunizations, such as measles, tetanus, and diphtheria vaccines. Approximately 20 million people have already died of HIV/AIDS over the past two decades. Forty million more are presently infected with HIV, and the virus continues to spread relentlessly, with its death toll reaching about 300 people every hour of the day. Currently, 2.4 billion people on the planet live at risk of contracting malaria. Each year 300 to 500 million contract the disease, and at least a million people die of it. Also on an annual basis, more than 8 million new cases of tuberculosis are diagnosed and 2 million people die of the white plague. And these are only some of the contagious threats facing humankind today. In the twenty-first century we live in a world where water supplies, food chains, social customs and practices, housing, and living conditions all impact everyone, eventually, whether we acknowledge it or not.[5]

At present, hundreds of thousands of men and women around the world devote their working lives and intellectual creativity to protecting our health. While they do a reasonably good job, given the resources they have at their command, many of them would readily admit that there is significant room for improvement. Not surprisingly, they are working under the same shadow that Abraham Cahan described in 1892: most people do not think much about putting precious resources into public health administration unless faced with a crisis.

Beyond the cultural differences that must be bridged in any international effort, combined with factors of national politics, priorities, and values, we continue to grapple with the essential paradox of public health that began our discussion: when the system is working effectively, it is a silent venture and there are relatively few outbreaks of disease. These very successes lead most of us down a complacent path of false confidence, apathy, and assumptions that the endless dance is over. To complicate matters further, microbes themselves are hardly monolithic or permanently settled beings. For every attempt we make to destroy or weaken them, they respond with an equal and opposite force. The goal of both sides is to assume leadership of the evolutionary waltz ever in progress.[6]

Epidemics have distinct contours and patterns of progression.[7] To begin with, someone needs to recognize and define the problem, and, as we have seen, this is not always such a simple task. It is always easier to declare an epidemic once the clinical scenario is better fleshed out. Most typically, a physician, health worker, or even careful observer notices that more people than usual in a particular community are developing a specific set of symptoms or a recognizable illness. Answers to many more questions that fit what epidemiologists call an "epi curve" must then augment these observations. How many new cases are there and precisely who is contracting it? What is the time frame of the appearance of new cases? Where is the illness striking and what are its geographical boundaries? What are the exact nature and cause of the disease? What organ systems are involved in the individuals with the ailment and how does it spread from person to person? Most important, how can it best be controlled given the technology of the day?

As with the 1900 bubonic plague epidemic in San Francisco's Chinatown, events can transpire from the local discovery of a deadly germ in one victim. In other cases, international epidemiological surveillance gives doctors advance warning of contagious diseases, as was the case with the physicians stationed at Ellis Island or along the Texas-Mexico border. More recently, laboratory methods have been applied including bacterial and viral cultures, RNA polymerase chain reaction (PCR) testing, antibody and immunoassay tests, and DNA and molecular fingerprint technologies that precisely identify the germ and the path it may have traveled around the world. All of these detection methods will play important roles in the dramas of humans and microbes unfolding today and tomorrow.

But when confronted with these crises, we must always recall Hermann Biggs's essential theorem of public health: it begins with the word "public." Imperious orders from on high, no matter how well intentioned, do not work well and often thwart efforts to safeguard health. A clearly marked plan of explanation, tolerance, education, and partnership between those orchestrating the battles against epidemics and the people who experience them firsthand is an absolute requirement to successful disease control. Scrupulous attention to the needs of the ill and their contacts is every bit as important as developing powerful antibiotics or vaccines and new means of international surveillance. While much has changed over the past century, our very human tendencies toward scapegoating or punishing the victim have not been completely eradicated and we must always be vigilant in keeping them in check.

As new diseases are discovered or old ones reappear, we should expect more false alarms, true crises, and dramatic announcements of infectious maladies that may or may not be great threats. Like the medical student who goes home convinced that he has the disease he has just learned about in the classroom that day, doctors and public health officials tend to overdiagnose illnesses that are in the news or latest medical journal. My diagnostic fiasco with cholera in Detroit is an excellent example of this.

Nothing less than a cooperative partnership of nations, health care professionals, researchers, public health specialists, concerned corporations, philanthropies, and individuals will suffice to safeguard the world against the many public health problems we face today. Dr. Biggs offered the best prescription for this ailment in 1911: "No duty of society, acting through its governmental agencies, is paramount to this obligation to attack the removable causes of disease." Much as a doctor can write a prescription, the patient must fill it and actually take the medicine. In this sense, we are all the patients, and all of us, from our leaders on down, must play our part in this lifesaving enterprise.

We can no longer ignore the urgent need to develop and support long-range, permanent prevention, surveillance, research, treatment, and educational public health strategies for everyone living in the world. To consider the health conditions of Africa or the former USSR or South America unimportant to those of Cleveland or Kansas City is beyond foolish; it will, inevitably, lead to disastrous consequences. As journalist Laurie Garrett recently observed, "global public health action on an ongoing basis would, if it truly existed, constitute disease prophylaxis for every locality, from rich nation to poor. . . . Safety, then, is as much a local as international issue. In public health terms, every city is a 'sister city' with every other metropolis on earth."[8] The explosion of AIDS in China and Africa and its robust presence in the United States, the resurgence of tuberculosis, cholera, malaria, typhus fever, and other "old-fashioned" plagues, the emergence of deadly microbes we are only beginning to recognize, and the potential for bioterrorist attacks all demonstrate that our responses to contagion are less than adequate. What makes this fact especially tragic is that we can actually do so much more to prevent and treat many of these scourges, provided we are prepared to make the necessary financial and social commitments to the task.[9]

In September 2000 the United Nations held a Millennium Summit where leaders of 180 different nations set several goals for promoting the health of all the world's citizens by the year 2015. Among these were controlling epidemic diseases, reducing the world's childhood mortality rate by 66 percent and the mortality rate of women during childbearing by 75 percent, reversing the global spread of HIV/AIDS, and halving the proportion of people in the world without access to safe drinking water or adequate food and whose income is less than one dollar a day.[10]

Columbia University economist Jeffrey Sachs was asked to develop a Commission on Macroeconomics and Health for the United Nations in order to chart a course for accomplishing these noble and lifesaving aims. The commission's three core findings were, first, that the massive amount of disease burden in the world's poorest nations poses a huge threat to global wealth and security. Second, millions of impoverished people around the world die of infectious diseases that are preventable and treatable because they lack access to medical care. And third, we have the ability and technology to save millions of lives each year if only the wealthier nations of the world would help provide the poorer countries with such health care and services.[11]

In terms of dollars and cents, this plan requires that all of the wealthy nations of the world devote at least one-tenth of one percent of their gross national product (or one penny for every ten dollars of income) toward supporting health services for the world's poor. For an average annual investment of $50 billion, coming from the world's high-income nations, we could prevent millions of child, maternal, and adult deaths annually. Think about it: 21,000 lives would be saved each day. And if the humane imperative is not enough, recall that with enhanced worldwide health, we also create vast improvements in the world economic picture due to more productive labor forces in nations currently decimated by disease. If we were to embark on this task today, the UN commission estimates that by 2020 more than $360 billion a year would be generated in other economic benefits.[12]

A more striking way to think about the cost of contributing to such a global public health effort is this: Sachs and his colleagues have estimated that if every person living in a high-income nation today denied him- or herself the luxury of one movie ticket and a bag of popcorn each year, the control of infectious killers such as AIDS, malaria, and tuberculosis could be easily funded at the levels recommended by the United Nations.[13]

We already have excellent evidence these endeavors can work. The global effort to eradicate smallpox through immunization programs of the world's poorest nations was a stunning success, even if it has been tarnished lately because of the threat of bioterrorism. Recent programs organized by a consortium of foundations, health agencies, and pharmaceutical companies to reduce or eliminate African river blindness, trachoma, AIDS, and leprosy in developing nations have been nothing short of miraculous. Yet each of these accomplishments constitutes a mere fraction of the work that not only human decency depends upon but also the basic survival of us all requires.

"Public health is purchasable," but it is an investment that works best when purchased in advance rather than paid out as each crisis arises. Germs travel in many ways, and the living beings that often carry them move widely about the world. This is not a trend likely to reverse itself, and all indications suggest it will only increase in magnitude. Regardless of one's political opinions about our nation's immigration policies or the suitability of newcomers to our shores, we must accept that contagion cannot be confined to national boundaries. The problem is far bigger than what the back of any social scapegoat can be expected to bear. The public's health is everybody's problem and responsibility, no matter where one comes from or lives. Only the global community can make inroads in safeguarding it, and even with the best of efforts, we will never completely conquer the microbial world.

NOTES

## INTRODUCTION

1. Leviticus 19:33–34.
2. Hans Zinsser, *Rats, Lice and History: Being a Study in Biography, Which After Twelve Preliminary Chapters Indispensable for the Preparation of the Lay Reader, Deals with the Life History of Typhus Fever* (Boston: Little, Brown, 1935), p. 7.
3. John F. Kennedy, *A Nation of Immigrants*, rev. and enl. ed. (New York: Harper-Collins, 1986); John Higham, *Strangers in the Land: Patterns of American Nativism, 1860–1925*, 2nd ed. (New Brunswick, N.J.: Rutgers University Press, 1988); Nancy Foner, *From Ellis Island to JFK: New York's Two Great Waves of Immigration* (New Haven: Yale University Press, 2000).
4. Howard Markel, *Quarantine!: East European Jewish Immigrants and the New York City Epidemics of 1892* (Baltimore: Johns Hopkins University Press, 1997), p. xiii.
5. Ruth Gay, *Unfinished People: Eastern European Jews Encounter America* (New York: Norton, 1996).
6. Charles Rosenberg, "What Is an Epidemic?: AIDS in Historical Perspective," in his *Explaining Epidemics and Other Studies in the History of Medicine* (New York: Cambridge University Press, 1992), pp. 278–92.
7. William Carlos Williams, *The Autobiography of William Carlos Williams* (New York: Random House, 1951), pp. 359–60. For another elegy by the same author on the power of these stories, see *A Beginning on the Short Story: Notes* (Yonkers, N.Y.: Alicat, 1950), pp. 5, 11, and *The Doctor Stories* (New York: New Directions, 1984). See also Sherwin Nuland, "Introduction," *The Collected Stories of William Carlos Williams* (New York: New Directions, 1996), pp. vii–xii.
8. Williams, *Autobiography*, p. 357.
9. Ibid., p. 391; Nuland, "Introduction," pp. vii–xii.

CHAPTER ONE • FACING TUBERCULOSIS

1. Abdul, interviewed by author, Columbia University Mailman School of Public Health, Oct. 12, 2001. All subsequent quotes from him are derived from this interview. I am indebted to Dr. Karen Brudney, the director of the New York–Presbyterian Hospital TB Clinic, for facilitating my interviews with Abdul and other tuberculosis patients.

2. Howard Markel, "Germ Culture," *Harper's*, March 2002, pp. 65–70; T. A. Mayer et al., "Clinical Presentation of Inhalational Anthrax Following Bioterrorism Exposure: Report of Two Surviving Patients," *Journal of the American Medical Association* 286 (2001): 2595–97; J. A. Jernigan et al., "Bioterrorism Related Inhalational Anthrax: The First 10 Cases Reported in the United States," *Emerging Infectious Diseases* 7 (2001): 933–44; L. M. Bush et al., "Index Case of Fatal Inhalational Anthrax Due to Bioterrorism in the United States," *New England Journal of Medicine* 345 (2001): 1607–10; Eric Lipton and Kirk Johnson, "Tracking Bioterror's Tangled Course: The Anthrax Trail," *New York Times*, Dec. 26, 2001, p. A1; Lawrence K. Altman and Gina Kolata, "Anthrax Missteps Offer Guide to Fight Next Bioterror Battle," *New York Times*, Jan. 6, 2002, p. A1.

3. Malcolm Gladwell, "Contagions: The Scourge You Know," *The New Yorker*, Oct. 29, 2001, pp. 33–34.

4. Quoted in René Dubos, *Louis Pasteur: Free Lance of Science* (New York: Scribner's, 1976), p. 45.

5. Paul Farmer, ed., *The Global Impact of Drug-Resistant Tuberculosis* (Boston: Harvard Medical School, 1999). See also World Health Organization, *Global Tuberculosis Control: WHO Reports for 2000, 2002, and 2003* (Geneva: World Health Organization, 2000–2003); Lawrence Geiter, ed., *Ending Neglect: The Elimination of Tuberculosis in the United States* (Washington, D.C.: National Academy Press, 2000); Lee B. Reichman and Janice Hopkins Tanne, *Timebomb: The Global Epidemic of Multidrug Resistant Tuberculosis* (New York: McGraw-Hill, 2002); "The Tuberculosis Threat," *New York Times*, July 19, 2001, p. A26; D. G. McNeil, "Resisting Drugs: TB Spreads Fast in the West," *New York Times*, Mar. 24, 2000, p. A10.

6. Alejandro, interview by author, Columbia University Mailman School of Public Health, Oct. 12, 2001. All subsequent quotes from him are derived from this interview.

7. Statement of Senator Carl Levin of Michigan speaking for the Permanent Subcommittee on Investigations Hearing on Release of Persons Arrested for Illegal Entry into the United States to the Senate Committee on Governmental Affairs, Nov. 13, 2001, http://govt-aff.senate.gov/111301levin.htm. Accessed Nov. 4, 2003; Ginger Thompson, "Mexico's Open Southern Border Lures Migrants Headed to U.S.," *New York Times*, Aug. 5, 2001, p. A1.

8. Judith Walzer Leavitt, *Typhoid Mary: Captive to the Public's Health* (Boston: Beacon, 1996); Anthony Bourdain, *Typhoid Mary: An Urban Historical* (New York: Bloomsbury, 2001).

9. Michael Iseman and Jeffrey Starke, "Immigrants and Tuberculosis Control," *New*

*England Journal of Medicine* 332 (1995): 1094–95; Tal Ann Ziv and Bernard Lo, "Denial of Care to Illegal Immigrants: Proposition 187 in California," *New England Journal of Medicine* 332 (1995): 1095–98; Steven Asch, Barbara Leake, and Lillian Gelberg, "Does Fear of Immigration Authorities Deter Tuberculosis Patients from Seeking Care?" *Western Journal of Medicine* 161 (1994): 373–76.

10. T. A. Kenyon et al., "Transmission of Multidrug-Resistant Mycobacterium Tuberculosis During a Long Airplane Flight," *New England Journal of Medicine* 334 (1996): 933–38; "Exposure of Passengers and Flight Crew to *Mycobacterium tuberculosis* on Commercial Aircraft, 1992–1995," *Morbidity and Mortality Weekly Report* 44 (1995): 137–40. See K. DeRiemer et al., "Tuberculosis Among Immigrants and Refugees," *Archives of Internal Medicine* 158 (1998): 753–60; M. T. McKenna, E. McCray, and I. Onorato, "The Epidemiology of Tuberculosis Among Foreign-Born Persons in the United States, 1986–1993," *New England Journal of Medicine* 332 (1995): 1071–76; J. Bayuk et al., "Tuberculosis Screening of Applicants for U.S. Immigration," *Journal of the American Medical Association* 273 (1995): 286–87; "News in Brief: WHO Warning for Air Passengers," *Lancet* 353 (1999): 305.

11. John Belisle and Patrick Brennan, "Mycobacteria," in *Encyclopedia of Microbiology,* 2nd ed., vol. 3, ed. Joshua Lederberg (San Diego: Academic Press, 2000), pp. 312–27; J. J. Adler and D. N. Rose, "Transmission and Pathogenesis of Tuberculosis," in *Tuberculosis,* ed. W. N. Rom and S. Garay (Boston: Little, Brown, 1996), pp. 129–40.

12. Arthur Vander, James Sherman, and Dorothy Luciano, *Human Physiology: The Mechanisms of Body Function* (New York: McGraw-Hill, 1994), pp. 474–76.

13. Judith Miller, Stephen Engelberg, and William Broad, *Germs: Biological Weapons and America's Secret War* (New York: Simon & Schuster, 2001), p. 43.

14. Michael Iseman, "Tuberculosis," in *Cecil Textbook of Medicine,* 21st ed., vol. 2 (Philadelphia: W. B. Saunders, 2000), pp. 1723–31; M. C. Raviglione and R. J. O'Brien, "Tuberculosis," in *Harrison's Principles of Internal Medicine,* 15th ed., vol. 1, ed. Eugene Braunwald et al. (New York: McGraw-Hill, 2001), pp. 1024–35.

15. Thomas Mann, *The Magic Mountain,* trans. John E. Woods (New York: Vintage, 1996).

16. Thomas Dormandy, *The White Death: A History of Tuberculosis* (New York: New York University Press, 2000), pp. 173–86; Barbara Bates, *Bargaining for Life: A Social History of Tuberculosis, 1876–1938* (Philadelphia: University of Pennsylvania Press, 1992), pp. 152–96.

17. Mann, *Magic Mountain,* 48–49. For the development of pneumothorax, see John Alexander, *The Surgery of Pulmonary Tuberculosis* (Philadelphia: Lea and Febiger, 1925), and *The Collapse Therapy of Pulmonary Tuberculosis* (Springfield, Ill.: C. C. Thomas, 1937); Ted Allan and Sydney Gordon, *The Scalpel, The Sword: The Story of Doctor Norman Bethune* (New York: Monthly Review Press, 1952). On recent uses of drastic lung surgery, see Lisa Belkin, "A Brutal Cure," *New York Times Magazine,* May 30, 1999, pp. 34–39.

18. Howard Markel, "The Death of Samuel Johnson, LL.D.: A Clinicopathologic Conference," *American Journal of Medicine* 82 (1987): 1203–7.

19. René Dubos and Jean Dubos, *The White Plague: Tuberculosis, Man and Society* (Boston: Little, Brown, 1952), pp. 3–10, 71–72.

20. Susan Sontag, *Illness as Metaphor* (New York: Farrar, Straus and Giroux, 1978), p. 13. See also Linda Hutcheon and Michael Hutcheon, *Opera: Desire, Disease, Death* (Lincoln: University of Nebraska Press, 1996); Lewis Moorman, *Tuberculosis and Genius* (Chicago: University of Chicago Press, 1940).

21. Claude E. Dolman, "Robert Koch," in *Dictionary of Scientific Biography,* vol. 7 (New York: Scribner's, 1973), pp. 420–33.

22. Abraham Jacobi, "Inaugural Address Delivered Before the New York Academy of Medicine, February 5, 1885," *Miscellaneous Addresses and Writings,* vol. 7 (New York: Critic and Guide, 1909), p. 170.

23. Louis Pasteur, "Inaugural Lecture, University of Lille, December 7, 1854," quoted in *Bartlett's Familiar Quotations,* 16th ed., ed. John Bartlett and Justin Kaplan (Boston: Little, Brown, 1992), p. 502.

24. Paul de Kruif, *Microbe Hunters* (New York: Harcourt, Brace, 1926), p. 336.

25. Lillian E. Prudden, ed., *Biographical Sketches and Letters of T. Mitchell Prudden, M.D.* (New Haven: Yale University Press, 1927).

26. T. Mitchell Prudden, *The Story of the Bacteria and Their Relations to Health and Disease* (New York: G. P. Putnam's Sons, 1889), *Dust and Its Dangers* (New York: G. P. Putnam's Sons, 1890), and *Drinking-Water and Ice Supplies* (New York: G. P. Putnam's Sons, 1891).

27. Prudden, *Dust and Its Dangers,* pp. 92–93.

28. Nancy Tomes, *The Gospel of Germs: Men, Women, and the Microbe in American Life* (Cambridge: Harvard University Press, 1998), p. 3.

29. Prudden, *Story of the Bacteria,* p. 75.

30. Prudden, *Dust and Its Dangers,* p. 97.

31. Tomes, *Gospel of Germs,* pp. 124, 194.

32. William Osler, *The Principles and Practices of Medicine* (New York: Appleton, 1892), p. 191; Prudden, *Story of the Bacteria,* p. 77.

33. W. F. Wells, *Airborne Contagion and Air Hygiene* (Cambridge: Harvard University Press, 1955). See also R. Riley and E. A. Nardell, "Clearing the Air: The Theory and Application of Ultraviolet Air Disinfection," *American Review of Respiratory Disease* 139 (1989): 1286–94. Also see R. Riley and F. O'Grady, *Airborne Infection* (New York: Macmillan, 1961). Also see E. A. Nardell, "Aerosol Infections," in *Encyclopedia of Microbiology,* 2nd ed., vol. 1, ed. Joshua Lederberg (San Diego: Academic Press, 2000), pp. 66–77.

34. Charles E. A. Winslow, *The Life of Hermann M. Biggs, M.D., D.Sc., LL.D.: Physician and Statesman of the Public Health* (Philadelphia: Lea and Febiger, 1929), pp. 131–52. See also Irving Howe, *World of Our Fathers: The Journey of the East European Jews to America and the Life They Found and Made* (New York: Harcourt Brace Jovanovich, 1976), pp. 149–50; Daniel Soyer, *Jewish Immigrant Associations and American Identity in New York, 1880–1939* (Cambridge: Harvard University Press, 1997).

35. (Mrs.) Prescott F. Hall, ed., *Immigration and Other Interests of Prescott Farnsworth Hall* (New York: Knickerbocker, 1922), p. xxv.

36. Prescott F. Hall, *Immigration and Its Effects upon the United States* (New York: Holt, 1906), p. 244.

37. Ibid.

38. Ibid., p. 85. On Hall's tuberculosis-immigrant connection, see also pp. 50, 158–59. For contemporary evidence on the paucity of tuberculosis among East European Jewish immigrants, see John Billings, "Vital Statistics of the Jews," *North American Review* 152 (1891): 70–85; Maurice Fishberg, *Health Problems of the Jewish Poor* [reprinted from *The American Hebrew*] (New York: Cowen, 1903).

39. Special Board of Inquiry Hearing Held at Ellis Island, New York Harbor for Supermoney Munsammy, Mar. 16, 1910, RG 85, Immigration and Naturalization Service (hereafter INS), Immigration Series Case Files, Box 230, Files 52880 (Acc. No. 60A/600), National Archives Records Administration, Washington, D.C.

40. Howard Markel, *Quarantine!: East European Jewish Immigrants and the New York City Epidemics of 1892* (Baltimore: Johns Hopkins University Press, 1997), p. 181. See also Daniel Kevles, *In the Name of Eugenics: Genetics and the Uses of Human Heredity* (New York: Knopf, 1985); Kenneth Ludmerer, *Genetics and American Society: A Historical Appraisal* (Baltimore: Johns Hopkins University Press, 1972); Garland Allen, "The Eugenics Record Office at Cold Spring Harbor, 1910–1940: An Essay in Institutional History," *OSIRIS* 2 (1986): 225–64; Barbara Miller Solomon, *Ancestors and Immigrants: A Changing New England Tradition* (Cambridge: Harvard University Press, 1956).

41. Hall, *Immigration and Other Interests,* p. 185.

42. Sheila Rothman, *Living in the Shadow of Death: Tuberculosis and the Social Experience of Illness in American History* (New York: Basic Books, 1994), pp. 211–41; Edward Livingston Trudeau, *An Autobiography* (Garden City, N.Y.: Doubleday, Page, 1916); David Ellison, *Healing Tuberculosis in the Woods: Medicine and Science at the End of the Nineteenth Century* (Westport, Ct.: Greenwood, 1994); Robert Taylor. *Saranac: America's Magic Mountain* (New York: Paragon House, 1986).

43. Georgina Feldberg, *Disease and Class: Tuberculosis and the Shaping of Modern North American Society* (New Brunswick, N.J.: Rutgers University Press, 1995), pp. 90–109; Bates, *Bargaining for Life,* pp. 135–314; Katherine Ott, *Fevered Lives: Tuberculosis in American Culture Since 1870* (Cambridge: Harvard University Press, 1996), pp. 69–86.

44. Dormandy, *White Death,* pp. 147–86. For a superb case history of the experience of tuberculosis during this period, one can hardly do better than to review the life and work of Eugene O'Neill. See Arthur Gelb and Barbara Gelb, *O'Neill: Life with Monte Cristo* (New York: Applause, 2000), pp. 369–93; Eugene O'Neill, *Long Day's Journey into Night* (New Haven: Yale University Press, 1955), and *The Straw,* in *The Emperor Jones, Diff'rent, The Straw* (New York: Boni and Liveright, 1921).

45. Leonard G. Wilson, "The Historical Decline of Tuberculosis in Europe and America," *Journal of the History of Medicine and Allied Sciences* 45 (1990): 366–96.

46. George Rosen, *A History of Public Health,* exp. ed. (Baltimore: Johns Hopkins University Press, 1993), pp. 361–66; Dubos, *White Plague,* pp. 172–81, 261–62.

47. Iva Marie Lowry, *Second Landing* (Philadelphia: Dorrance, 1974), p. 53.

48. William Osler, "Teaching and Thinking: The Two Functions of a Medical School," in *Aequanimitas with Other Addresses to Medical Students* (Philadelphia: Blakiston, 1904), p. 131.

49. Selman Waksman, *My Life with the Microbes* (New York: Simon & Schuster, 1954).

50. Brent Hoff and Carter Smith III, "Tuberculosis," in *Mapping Epidemics: A Historical Atlas of Disease* (New York: Watts/Grolier, 2000), p. 94.

51. Waksman, *My Life with the Microbes*, p. 235; Dubos, *White Plague*, pp. 154-72.

52. Geiter, *Ending Neglect*, p. 17.

53. Evan Charney et al., "How Well Do Patients Take Oral Penicillin?: A Collaborative Study in Private Practice," *Pediatrics* 40 (1967): 188-95; A. B. Bergman and R. J. Werner, "Failure of Children to Receive Penicillin by Mouth," *New England Journal of Medicine* 268 (1963): 1334-38.

54. Farmer, *Global Impact of Drug-Resistant Tuberculosis*, p. xiii. See also Geiter, *Ending Neglect*, p. 17; M. A. Espinal et al., "Global Trends in Resistance to Antituberculosis Drugs," *New England Journal of Medicine* 344 (2001): 1294-1303; M. Lipsitch, R. Singer, and B. Levin, "Antibiotics in Agriculture: When Is It Time to Close the Barn Door?" *Proceedings of the National Academy of Sciences* 99 (2002): 5752-54.

55. Karen Brudney and Jay Dobkin, "Resurgent Tuberculosis in New York City," *American Review of Respiratory Disease* 144 (1991): 745-49, and "A Tale of Two Cities: Tuberculosis Control in Nicaragua and New York City," *Seminars in Respiratory Infections* 6 (1991): 261-72.

56. Reichman and Hopkins Tanne, *Timebomb*, p. 143.

57. Brudney and Dobkin, "Resurgent Tuberculosis in New York City," and Thomas R. Frieden et al., "Tuberculosis in New York City: Turning the Tide," *New England Journal of Medicine* 333 (1995): 229-33, and "The Emergence of Drug-Resistant Tuberculosis in New York City," *New England Journal of Medicine* 328 (1993): 521-26.

58. Reichman and Hopkins Tanne, *Timebomb*, pp. 145-54.

59. Ibid., p. 154.

60. Elvin Geng et al., "Changes in the Transmission of Tuberculosis in New York City from 1990 to 1999," *New England Journal of Medicine* 346 (2002): 1453-58; Barry Bloom, "Tuberculosis: The Global View," *New England Journal of Medicine* 346 (2002): 1434-35.

61. Bloom, "Tuberculosis," pp. 1434-35. For a report on the recent success in controlling tuberculosis in India by means of improving access to care, the quality of diagnosis, and the likelihood of effective treatment, see G. R. Khatri and Thomas R. Frieden, "Controlling Tuberculosis in India," *New England Journal of Medicine* 347 (2002): 1420-25; Jeffrey Drazen, "A Milestone in Tuberculosis Control," *New England Journal of Medicine* 347 (2002): 1444.

CHAPTER TWO • BUBONIC PLAGUE VISITS SAN FRANCISCO'S CHINATOWN

1. *San Francisco Chronicle*, Mar. 8, 1900, p. 7.

2. The sources for this section include Ann Carmichael, "Plague," in *The Cambridge*

*World History of Human Disease,* ed. Kenneth Kiple (New York: Cambridge University Press, 1993), pp. 628–31, and *Plague and the Poor in Renaissance Florence* (Cambridge, Eng.: Cambridge University Press, 1986); David Herlihy, *The Black Death and the Transformation of the West* (Cambridge: Harvard University Press, 1997); Paul Slack, "The Black Death Past and Present: Some Historical Problems," *Transactions of the Royal Society of Tropical Medicine and Hygiene* 83 (1989): 461–63; Leonard Fabian Hirst, *The Conquest of Plague: A Study of the Evolution of Epidemiology* (Oxford, Eng.: Clarendon, 1953); Geddes Smith, *Plague on Us* (New York: Commonwealth Fund, 1941); Norman Cantor, *In the Wake of the Plague: The Black Death and the World It Made* (New York: Free Press, 2001); George Rosen, *A History of Public Health* (New York: MD Publications, 1958), pp. 43–45; Susan Scott and Christopher Duncan, *Biology of Plagues: Evidence from Historical Populations* (Cambridge, Eng.: Cambridge University Press, 2001); Guy Cornelis, "Molecular and Cell Biology Aspects of Plague," *Proceedings of the National Academy of Sciences* 97 (2000): 8778–83; J. Parkhill et al., "Genome Sequence of *Yersinia Pestis,* the Causative Agent of Plague," *Nature* 413 (2001): 523–27; Stewart Cole and Carmen Buchrieser, "Bacterial Genomics: A Plague o' Both Your Hosts," *Nature* 413 (2001): 467–70; Nicholas Wade, "DNA Map for Bacterium of Plague Is Decoded," *New York Times,* Oct. 4, 2001, p. A9; M. J. Keeling and C. A. Gilligan, "Metapopulation Dynamics of Bubonic Plague," *Nature* 407 (2000): 903–6; W. J. Calvert, "Plague," in *Osler's Modern Medicine,* vol. 2, ed. William Osler (New York: Lea and Febiger, 1907), pp. 760–80; Colin McEvedy, "The Bubonic Plague," *Scientific American* 258 (1988): 118–23; R. D. Perry and J. D. Fetherston, "*Yersinia Pestis:* Etiologic Agent of Plague," *Clinical Microbiology Reviews* 10 (1997): 35–66; T. V. Inglesby et al., "Plague as a Biological Weapon: Medical and Public Health Management," *Journal of the American Medical Association* 283 (2000): 2281–90.

3. Jacob Riis, *How the Other Half Lives: Studies Among the Tenements of New York* (New York: Scribner's, 1890), pp. 87–88.

4. Chick Gin is also referred to as Wing Chung Ging or Wong Chut King in the contemporary press. I chose to use the name Chick Gin because it appeared most often in the daily editions of the *San Francisco Chronicle.* The Chick Gin case is primarily drawn from newspaper accounts in the *San Francisco Chronicle, San Francisco Examiner, San Francisco Call,* and *Sacramento Bee,* Mar. 6–10, 1900. See Philip Kalisch, "The Black Death in Chinatown: Plague and Politics in San Francisco, 1900–1904," *Journal of the Southwest* 14 (1972): 113–36; Charles McClain, *In Search of Equality: The Chinese Struggle Against Discrimination in Nineteenth-Century America* (Berkeley: University of California Press, 1994), pp. 234–76. This source is especially helpful because of the inclusion of translated articles from the Chinese press in its text. See also Alan Kraut, *Silent Travelers: Germs, Genes, and the "Immigrant Menace"* (New York: Basic Books, 1994), pp. 78–96; Nayan Shah, *Contagious Divides: Epidemics and Race in San Francisco's Chinatown* (Berkeley: University of California Press, 2001), pp. 120–57; Howard Zentner, *Human Plague in the United States from 1900 to 1940* (New Orleans: Tulane University Press, 1942); Vernon Link, *A History of Plague in the United States of America* (Washington, D.C.: U.S. Government Printing Office, 1955); Joan Trauner, "The Chinese as

Medical Scapegoats in San Francisco, 1870–1905," *California Historical Quarterly* 57 (1978): 70–87.

5. Sherwin Nuland, *The Mysteries Within: A Surgeon Reflects on Medical Myths, Medicine, and the Human Body* (New York: Simon & Schuster, 2000).

6. A recent and wonderfully engaging account of plague in San Francisco, Marilyn Chase, *The Barbary Plague: The Black Death in Victorian San Francisco* (New York: Random House, 2003), traces the importation of *Yersinia* into San Francisco in 1900 to one steamship, the S.S. *Australia*, but it remains difficult to verify such a precise event; Felix Riesenberg Jr., *Golden Gate: The Story of San Francisco Harbor* (New York: Knopf, 1940), p. 247; Ronald Takaki, *Strangers from a Different Shore: A History of Asian Americans* (Boston: Little, Brown, 1989).

7. Kil Young Zo, *Chinese Emigration into the United States, 1850–1880* (New York: Arno, 1978), pp. 54–79; Cheng-Tsu Wu, ed., *Chink!: A Documentary History of Anti-Chinese Prejudice in America* (New York: World, 1972); Sucheng Chan, *Asian Americans: An Interpretive History* (Boston: Twayne, 1991), pp. 5–7; William Hoy, *The Chinese Six Companies* (San Francisco: Chinese Consolidated Benevolent Association, 1942), p. 16. In point of fact, almost all the Chinese immigrants coming to the United States during the nineteenth and early twentieth centuries originated from the Hsin-ning (Four Towns) district and its surrounding districts of Hsin-hui, K'ai-p'ing, and Enp'ing; this area was known collectively as Sze-Yap. The other nearby source of Chinese immigration included the Pearl River district, which included the city of Canton.

8. Mary Roberts Coolidge, *Chinese Immigration* (New York: Henry Holt, 1909), p. 98; Helen Chen, "Chinese Immigration into the United States: An Analysis of Changes in Immigration Policies" (Ph.D. diss., Brandeis University, 1980), pp. 175–91.

9. Coolidge, *Chinese Immigration*, pp. 279, 504; Delber McKee, *Chinese Exclusion Versus the Open Door Policy, 1900–1906: Clashes over China Policy in the Roosevelt Era* (Detroit: Wayne State University Press, 1977), pp. 15–51.

10. Edward Ross, *The Old World in the New* (New York: Century, 1914), p. 226; Lucy Salyer, *Laws Harsh as Tigers: Chinese Immigrants and the Shaping of Modern Immigration Law* (Chapel Hill: University of North Carolina Press, 1995); Andrew Gyory, *Closing the Gate: Race, Politics, and the Chinese Exclusion Act* (Chapel Hill: University of North Carolina Press, 1998).

11. Walter Wyman, *The Bubonic Plague* (Washington, D.C.: U.S. Government Printing Office, 1900), pp. 7–9; Carol Benedict, *Bubonic Plague in Nineteenth-Century China* (Stanford: Stanford University Press, 1996); William McNeill, *Plagues and People* (Garden City, N.Y.: Anchor, 1976).

12. *Honolulu Bulletin*, Dec. 19, 1899, 1:1; *Pacific Commercial Advertiser*, Dec. 13, 1899, pp. 1–3, 9; Dec. 15, 1899, pp. 1, 4; Dec. 16, 1899, pp. 1, 5; Dec. 18, 1899, p. 1. See telegrams from Surgeon Kinyoun to General Wyman, Jan. 20, 1900, Feb. 1, 10, 1900, RG 90, box 552, National Archives Records Administration, College Park, Md. Major Ruhlen to General Wyman, typescript of telephone message, Feb. 15, 1900, RG 90, box 561, National Archives Records Administration; *San Francisco Chronicle*, Mar. 10, 1900, p. 4.

13. Chick Gin's confusing, and at times contradictory, medical history is drawn from reports in *San Francisco Chronicle,* Mar. 9, 1900, p. 1; *San Francisco Examiner,* Mar. 9, 1900, p. 1; *San Francisco Call,* Mar. 9, 1900, 12:1.

14. For the history of Chinese immigration to the United States via Mexican and Canadian borders during this period, see Erika Lee, "Enforcing the Borders: Chinese Exclusion Along the U.S. Borders with Canada and Mexico, 1882–1924," *Journal of American History* 89 (2002): 54–86. For background on the Chinese prostitution trade in San Francisco, see Judy Yung, *Unbound Feet: A Social History of Chinese Women in San Francisco* (Berkeley: University of California Press, 1995), pp. 71–72.

15. *San Francisco Chronicle,* Mar. 8, 1900, p. 7.

16. Hirst, *Conquest of Plague,* pp. 152–88; Robert Koch, *Essays of Robert Koch,* trans. K. Codell Carter (New York: Greenwood, 1987).

17. During his years in Washington, Kinyoun also managed to complete a Ph.D. at Georgetown University in 1896. For biographical information on Kinyoun, see Joseph Kinyoun Papers, box 1, files 1–15, History of Medicine Division, National Library of Medicine, Bethesda, Md.; Ralph Williams, *The United States Public Health Service, 1798–1950* (Washington, D.C.: Commissioned Officers Association of the United States Public Health Service, 1951), pp. 176–81, 249–50; Paul Clark, *Pioneer Microbiologists of America* (Madison: University of Wisconsin Press, 1961), pp. 206–7; Victoria Harden, *Inventing the NIH: Federal Biomedical Research Policy, 1887–1937* (Baltimore: Johns Hopkins University Press, 1986), pp. 12–15; Hermann M. Biggs, "The Diagnostic Value of the Cholera Spirillum as Illustrated by the Investigation of a Case at the New York Quarantine Station," *New York Medical Journal* 46 (1887): 548–49.

18. *San Francisco Chronicle,* Mar. 13, 1900, p. 12. For articles documenting "no results yet" at Angel Island, see *San Francisco Examiner,* Mar. 9, 1900, p. 9; *San Francisco Chronicle,* Mar. 10, 1900, p. 7; *San Francisco Call,* Mar. 10, 1900, p. 12.

19. *San Francisco Chronicle,* Mar. 12, 1900, p. 7.

20. Yong Chen, *Chinese San Francisco, 1850–1943: A Trans-Pacific Community* (Stanford: Stanford University Press, 2000); Riesenberg, *Golden Gate,* pp. 162–63; Carol Wilson, *Chinatown Quest: The Life Adventures of Donaldina Cameron* (Stanford: Stanford University Press, 1931); Takaki, *Strangers from a Different Shore,* pp. 239–57.

21. *San Francisco Chronicle,* Mar. 8, 1900, p. 7.

22. The Highbinders (secret Chinese gangs known for extorting money and killing merchants) were widely reported in the San Francisco press. See, for example, "Gunfighters of See Yup Tong, Go Forth to Shoot and Kill," *San Francisco Chronicle,* Mar. 6, 1900, p. 12.

23. *San Francisco Chronicle,* Mar. 8, 1900, p. 7; *San Francisco Examiner,* Mar. 8, 1900, p. 6.

24. *Chung Sai Yat Po,* Mar. 8, 1900, p. 1, quoted in McClain, *In Search of Equality,* p. 237. See also *San Francisco Examiner,* Mar. 8, 1900, p. 7.

25. *San Francisco Examiner,* Mar. 9, 1900, p. 9.

26. *San Francisco Examiner,* Mar. 8, 1900, p. 7.

27. *San Francisco Chronicle*, Mar. 10, 1900, p. 7.

28. Ibid.; *San Francisco Call*, Mar. 11, 1900, p. 19.

29. *San Francisco Call*, Mar. 13, 1900, p. 4.

30. *San Francisco Examiner*, Mar. 18, 1900, p. 7.

31. *San Francisco Examiner*, Mar. 23, 1900, p. 7.

32. *Sacramento Record-Union*, Mar. 23, 1900, p. 6; *San Francisco Call*, Mar. 27, 1900, p. 1.

33. *San Francisco Examiner*, Mar. 13, 1900, p. 7.

34. For the California campaign to assure the nation that all was under control, see *San Francisco Chronicle*, Mar. 24, 1900. For Wyman's response to the situation, see *Annual Report of the Supervising Surgeon General of the U.S. Marine Hospital Service, for 1900–1901* (Washington, D.C.: U.S. Government Printing Office, 1901), p. 538. All of these telegrams between Wyman and his assistant surgeons during the 1900 epidemic are reprinted in this annual report, pp. 530–71. The originals can be found at the National Archives Records Administration, RG 90, United States Public Health Service (hereafter USPHS) Bubonic Plague, San Francisco, 1900.

35. *Annual Report of the Supervising Surgeon General, 1900–1901*, p. 539.

36. Howard Markel, *Quarantine!: East European Jewish Immigrants and the New York City Epidemics of 1892* (Baltimore: Johns Hopkins University Press, 1997), pp. 179–82. See also Alan Marcus, "Disease Prevention in America: From a Local to a National Outlook, 1880–1910," *Bulletin of the History of Medicine* 53 (1979): 184–203; Margaret Humphreys, *Yellow Fever and the South* (New Brunswick, N.J.: Rutgers University Press, 1992); Hugh Cumming, "The United States Quarantine System During the Last Fifty Years," in *A Half Century of Public Health*, ed. Mazyck P. Ravenel (New York: American Public Health Association, 1921), pp. 118–32; James Tobey, *The National Government and Public Health* (Baltimore: Johns Hopkins University Press, 1926).

37. For an example of how patronage politics and commercial interests obstructed public health matters in San Francisco around this period, see *Annual Report of the Supervising Surgeon General of the U.S. Marine Health Service for 1897* (Washington, D.C.: U.S. Government Printing Office, 1898), p. 503.

38. U.S. Marine Hospital Service, *Department Circular No. 93*, May 22, 1900; *Annual Report of the Supervising Surgeon General 1900–1901*, pp. 530–71; Charles McClain, "Of Medicine, Race, and American Law: The Bubonic Plague Outbreak of 1900," *Law and Social Inquiry* 13 (1988): 447–513.

39. Shah, *Contagious Divides*, pp. 133–39.

40. Coolidge, *Chinese Immigration*, p. 402.

41. Both the Six Companies petition and the MacGuire quote are from *San Francisco Examiner*, June 1, 1900, p. 6.

42. Ibid., p. 3.

43. *San Francisco Examiner*, June 3, 1900, p. 6.

44. *San Francisco Examiner*, June 2, 1900, p. 3. See also *Sacramento Bee*, June 1, 1900, p. 1.

45. *San Francisco Examiner*, June 2, 1900, p. 3.

46. *Annual Report of the Supervising Surgeon General, 1900–1901*, pp. 562–63.

47. *San Francisco Examiner,* June 4, 1900, p. 6; June 5, 1900, p. 3.

48. *San Francisco Examiner,* June 5, 1900, p. 3.

49. W. M. W. Haffkine, "Remarks on the Plague Prophylactic Fluid," *British Medical Journal* 1 (1897): 461. See also Selman Waksman, *The Brilliant and Tragic Life of W. M. W. Haffkine, Bacteriologist* (New Brunswick, N.J.: Rutgers University Press, 1964), pp. 30–52, 61–67; J. Taylor, "Haffkine's Plague Vaccine," *Indian Journal of Medical Research (Indian Medical Research Memoirs)* 27 (1933): 1–9.

50. *Chung Sai Yat Po,* May 18, 1900, quoted in McClain, *In Search of Equality,* p. 247.

51. Six Companies and Ho Yow to Chinese Minister, telegram, May 19, 1900, RG 90, Bubonic Plague, San Francisco, 1900, National Archives Records Administration. The Chinese minister passed this cable on to Surgeon General Wyman with the request that his officers use "more tact and discretion so as to avoid complications." *Sacramento Record-Union,* May 22, 1900, p. 1.

52. *San Francisco Examiner,* June 7, 1900, p. 3.

53. *San Francisco Examiner,* June 11, 1900, p. 11.

54. *San Francisco Examiner,* June 10, 1900, p. 34.

55. *Wong Wai v. Williamson,* 103 F. 1,4 and 1,5 (C.C.N.D. Cal 1900); *Jew Ho v. Williamson,* 103 F. 10, 16–17 (C.C.N.D. Cal 1900); *Wong Wai v. Williamson,* Civil Case No. 12, 937, RG 21, National Archives, Pacific-Sierra Regional Branch at San Bruno, CA. For a superb legal analysis of these proceedings, see McClain, *In Search of Equality,* pp. 265–76; Alan Kraut, *Silent Travelers,* p. 92. The landmark case of a court supporting a health official's legal authority to order compulsory vaccinations was decided by the U.S. Supreme Court in 1905. See *Jacobson v. Massachusetts,* 197 U.S. 11, 25 S.Ct. 358 (1905).

56. *San Francisco Chronicle,* June 17, 1900, p. 11; June 19, 1900, pp. 6, 9; July 3, 1900, p. 12; July 4, 1900, p. 8; *San Francisco Examiner,* June 17, 1900, p. 15; June 19, 1900, p. 8; July 3, 1900, p. 7; July 4, 1900, p. 12; the cartoon appeared in *Chung Sai Yat Po,* June 22, 1900, p. 1.

57. Ralph Williams, *The United States Public Health Service, 1798–1950* (Washington, D.C.: Commissioned Officers Association of the United States Public Health Service, 1951), pp. 249–50; Joseph Kinyoun Papers, MS C 464, History of Medicine Division, National Library of Medicine. I am grateful to Robert Barde of the University of California at Berkeley for sharing his Kinyoun and Angel Island materials with me.

58. *San Francisco Examiner,* June 16, 1900, p. 5; *San Francisco Chronicle,* July 4, 1900, p. 8; July 5, 1900, p. 6; July 6, 1900, p. 4; *Sacramento Bee,* Aug. 15, 1900, p. 1; Oct. 16, 1900, p. 1; Nov. 10, 1900, p. 1; Nov. 15, 1900, p. 7; Dec. 11, 1900, p. 2.

59. The three plague experts were Frederick Novy, professor of bacteriology at the University of Michigan; Lewellys Barker, professor of medicine at the University of Chicago; and Simon Flexner, scientific director of the Rockefeller Institute. *Report of the Commission Appointed by the Secretary of the Treasury for the Investigation of Plague in San Francisco Under the Instructions from the Surgeon-General, Marine-Hospital Service* (Washington, D.C.: U.S. Government Printing Office, 1901).

60. Sinclair Lewis, *Arrowsmith* (New York: Harcourt, Brace, 1925); Paul de Kruif, *The*

*Sweeping Wind: A Memoir* (New York: Harcourt, Brace and World, 1962), and *From Main Street to Stockholm: Letters of Sinclair Lewis, 1919–1930*, ed. Harrison Smith (New York: Harcourt, Brace, 1952), pp. 121–89; Howard Markel, "Prescribing *Arrowsmith*," *New York Times Book Review*, Sept. 28, 2000, p. 35. See also George Dock, Apr. 26, 1901, Clinical Notebooks of George Dock, M.D., Professor of Medicine at the University of Michigan, vol. 2, Bentley Historical Library, University of Michigan, pp. 783–803; Frederick Novy Papers, Bubonic Plague File, Bentley Historical Library; W. A. Benscoter, "Ann Arbor's Case of Bubonic Plague," *Detroit News-Tribune*, Apr. 12, 1901, p. 2; Horace Davenport, *Not Just Any Medical School: The Science, Practice, and Teaching of Medicine at the University of Michigan, 1850–1941* (Ann Arbor: University of Michigan Press, 1999), p. 46; J. G. Cumming, "The Plague: A Laboratory Case Report," *Military Medicine* 128 (1963): 435–39; Mark Schorer, *Sinclair Lewis: An American Life* (New York: McGraw-Hill, 1961); Richard Lingeman, *Sinclair Lewis: Rebel from Main Street* (New York: Random House, 2002).

61. "Plague Investigations in India," *Public Health Reports* 22 (1907): 1799–1817; Frank Morton Todd, *Eradicating Plague from San Francisco: Report of the Citizen's Health Committee, March 31, 1909* (San Francisco: Murdock, 1909), pp. 19–24, 55–56; C. A. Gill, "The Epidemiology of Plague," *Lancet* 1 (1908): 213–16; Rupert Blue, "Plague in California and the Anti-Plague Campaign," *Journal of the American Medical Association* 51 (1908): 1010–14; G. W. McCoy, "The Extermination of Rats for Plague Infection," *Military Medicine* 24 (1909): 538–44; Guenter Risse, "A Long Pull, A Strong Pull, and All Together: San Francisco and Bubonic Plague, 1907–1908," *Bulletin of the History of Medicine* 66 (1992): 260–86; Marilyn Chase, *The Barbary Plague: The Black Death in Victorian San Francisco* (New York: Random House, 2003); Arthur Viseltear, "The Pneumonic Plague Epidemic of 1924 in Los Angeles," *Yale Journal of Biology and Medicine* 47 (1974): 40–54; W. Deverell, "Plague in Los Angeles, 1924: Ethnicity and Typicality," in *Over the Edge: Remapping the American West*, ed. V. J. Matsumoto and B. Allmendinger (Berkeley: University of California Press, 1999), pp. 172–200; Laurie Garrett, *Betrayal of Trust: The Collapse of Global Public Health* (New York: Hyperion, 2000), pp. 24–49.

62. Thomas Lueck, "New Mexico Man Seriously Ill with Plague in New York," *New York Times*, Nov. 7, 2002, p. A26; Cecelia Vega and Tina Kelley, "Couple Remain Hospitalized with Bubonic Plague," *New York Times*, Nov. 9, 2002, p. A17; Cecelia Vega, "One Plague Patient Is Released," *New York Times*, Nov. 14, 2002, p. B12; Anthony DePalma, "Plague Left a Man on the Brink, a City on Edge," *New York Times*, Feb. 7, 2003, p. A24; K. L. Gage, "Plague," in *Topley and Wilson's Microbiology and Microbial Infections*, vol. 3, ed. Colliers et al. (London: Arnold, 1998), pp. 885–903.

63. "Plague in Perspective," *New York Times*, Nov. 8, 2002, p. A32; "Samples of Bubonic Plague Stolen from Texas Tech," *CNN Breaking News*, Jan. 15, 2003, Transcript # 011503CN.V00; Russell Gold, "With Plague Fears on Rise, An Expert Ends Up on Trial," *Wall Street Journal*, Apr. 14, 2003, p. A1; See also Ed Regis, *The Biology of Doom: The History of America's Secret Germ Warfare Project* (New York: Henry Holt, 1999), pp. 3–6; Judith Miller, Stephen Engelberg, and William

Broad, *Germs: Biological Weapons and America's Secret War* (New York: Simon & Schuster, 2001), pp. 34–65.

64. Albert Camus, *The Plague*, trans. Stuart Gilbert (New York: Vintage International, 1991), p. 308.

### CHAPTER THREE • THE RABBI WITH TRACHOMA:
### THE VIEW FROM ELLIS ISLAND

1. Fiorello La Guardia, *The Making of an Insurgent: An Autobiography, 1882–1919* (Philadelphia: Lippincott, 1948), pp. 64–65. For historical accounts of the trachoma examinations, see Alan Kraut, *Silent Travelers: Germs, Genes, and the "Immigrant Menace"* (New York: Basic Books, 1994); Elizabeth Yew, "Medical Inspection of Immigrants at Ellis Island, 1891–1924," *Bulletin of the New York Academy of Medicine* 56 (1980): 488–510; Anne-Emanuelle Birn, "Six Seconds Per Eyelid: The Medical Inspection of Immigrants at Ellis Island, 1892–1914," *Dynamis* 17 (1997): 281–316; Howard Markel, "The Eyes Have It: Trachoma, the Perception of Disease, the U.S. Public Health Service, and the American Jewish Immigration Experience, 1897–1924," *Bulletin of the History of Medicine* 74 (2000): 525–60.

2. The experiences of Rabbi Goldenbaum are drawn from his case file in the Hebrew Immigrant Aid Society Collection, Ellis Island Bureau, 1905–1923, YIVO Institute, New York (microfilm MK10.8) and his case file at the U.S. INS (Card #3232257/Case #164101), Washington, D.C. See also the ship's manifest of the *S.S. San Guglielmo, Passenger and Crew List of Vessels Arriving at New York, 1887–1942* (Sept. 19, 25, 1916), vol. 5785–87, National Archives Records Administration, Washington, D.C. (microfilm T-715 #2490).

3. See, for example, Broughton Brandenberg, *Imported Americans* (New York: Stokes, 1904), pp. 138–39, 166–70, 200–201, 216–17; Arthur Henry, "Among the Immigrants," *Scribner's Magazine* 29 (1901): 301–11; Allan McLaughlin, "Immigration and the Public Health," *Popular Science Monthly* 64 (1903): 232–38, "The Problem of Immigration," *Popular Science Monthly* 65 (1905): 531–37, and "How Immigrants Are Inspected," *Popular Science Monthly* 65 (1905): 357–61; Alfred C. Reed, "Immigration and the Public Health," *Popular Science Monthly* 83 (1913): 320–38, and "Going Through Ellis Island," *Popular Science Monthly* 82 (1913): 5–18.

4. "Health Specialists Find Children's Eyes Diseased," *New York Times*, July 31, 1902, 9:6; "Emergency Hospital for Treatment of Trachoma," *New York Times*, Jan. 25, 1903, part 3, 25:1–2; H. W. Wooton, "The Treatment of Trachoma in School Children and the Clinical Features of the Disease," *Monthly Bulletin of the Department of Health of the City of New York* 1 (1911): 79–81; S. J. Baker, "The Control of Trachoma in School Children," *Monthly Bulletin of the Department of Health of the City of New York* 1 (1911): 82–84.

5. For allocation of financial and human resources by the USPHS during this period, see *Annual Reports of the Surgeon General of the U.S. Public Health Service and Marine Hospital Service, 1897–1924* (Washington, D.C.: U.S. Government Print-

ing Office, 1897–1924). The U.S. Marine Hospital Service became the U.S. Marine Hospital and Public Health Service in 1902. In 1912, it formally became the U.S. Public Health Service.

6. La Guardia, *Making of an Insurgent,* pp. 64–65.

7. See, for example, David Brownstone, Irene Franck, and Douglass Brownstone, eds., *Island of Hope, Island of Tears* (New York: Rawson Wade, 1979); Harlan Unrau, *Ellis Island, Statue of Liberty National Monument,* vol. 2 (Washington, D.C.: U.S. Department of the Interior/National Park Service, 1984), pp. 575–732.

8. Quoted in Charles May, *Manual of the Diseases of the Eye for Students and General Practitioners,* 6th ed. (New York: William Wood, 1909), p. 97. See also Louis Julianelle, *The Etiology of Trachoma* (New York: Oxford University Press, 1938); D. W. Vastine et al., "Severe Endemic Trachoma in Tunisia: Effect of Topical Chemotherapy on Conjunctivitis and Ocular Bacteria," *British Journal of Ophthalmology* 58 (1974): 833–42; P. Courtright et al., "Trachoma and Blindness in the Nile Delta: Current Patterns and Projections for the Future in the Rural Egyptian Population," *British Journal of Ophthalmology* 73 (1989): 536–40.

9. Conference to Consider Medical Examination of Immigrants Convened by Oscar Straus, Secretary of Commerce and Labor, Feb. 8, 1907, INS, Subject Correspondence, 1906–1932, file 51490/19, RG 85, National Archives Records Administration, Washington, D.C.; minutes of the National Jewish Immigration Committee, Mar. 13, 1912, Collections of the American Jewish Historical Society, Waltham, Mass.

10. Special Board of Inquiry pertaining to Sara Kupferman, case #98542/205, INS 60A/600 Collection, box 398, file 53370/143, RG 85, National Archives Records Administration.

11. Exact statistics from the Public Health and Immigration Services are difficult to assess because of the frequent change of categories from year to year and different numbers used for the same issue in the same reports. This figure was reached by surveying the *Annual Report of the Commissioner General of Immigration to the Secretary of Labor* (Washington, D.C.: U.S. Government Printing Office, 1900–1905).

12. William Williams to the Commissioner General of Immigration, Apr. 29, 1910, Special Board of Inquiry pertaining to Ruth Selkridge, INS Collection 60A/600, box 76, file 2, RG 85, National Archives Records Administration.

13. John A. McMullan, "A Report on an Investigation of the Prevalence of Trachoma in the Mountains of Eastern Kentucky," *Public Health Reports* 27 (1912): 1815–22. Quote is from p. 1818.

14. For studies of the trachoma problem among American Indians, see William Harrison, *Trachoma: Its Cause, Prevention and Treatment* (Washington, D.C.: U.S. Government Printing Office, 1915); J. W. Schereschewsky, "Trachoma Among the Indians," *Journal of the American Medical Association* 61 (1913): 1113–16; "Trachoma in Certain Indian Schools," *U.S. Senate Report No. 1025,* 60th Congr., 2nd sess., Feb. 18, 1909 (Washington, D.C.: U.S. Government Printing Office, 1909). Native Americans living in Oklahoma, Wyoming, Nebraska, Utah, Arizona, and New Mexico suffered the highest rates of trachoma.

15. For a discussion of the concept of infection and contagion, see Owsei Temkin, "An Historical Analysis of the Concept of Infection," in his *The Double Face of Janus and Other Essays in the History of Medicine* (Baltimore: Johns Hopkins University Press, 1977).

16. Dr. Walter S. Wyman to Frank H. Larned, October 30, 1897, *Copies of Letters Sent by the Office of the Surgeon General, 1872–1918,* vol. 137, pp. 303–304, RG 90, National Archives, College Park, Md. See also Myles Standish, "Contagious Conjunctivitis," *Boston Medical and Surgical Journal* 137, no. 6 (1897):129–31. Standish, a descendant of the Mayflower immigrant bearing the same name, was a Boston ophthalmologist who provided the expert testimony upon which Wyman based his trachoma circular of 1897.

17. Regulations pertaining to the inspection for and handling of immigrants with trachoma became more rigid and standardized with the passage of the Immigration Act of 1907, which specified that the Public Health Service certify all immigrants with mental and/or physical defects "which may affect the ability of such an alien to earn a living." Feb. 20, 1907, c. 1134, 34 Stat. 898. See E. P. Hutchinson, *Legislative History of American Immigration Policy, 1798–1965* (Philadelphia: University of Pennsylvania Press, 1981), pp. 85–196; *Reports of the Immigration Commission: Emigration Conditions in Europe,* vol. 4, U.S. Senate Document #748, 61st Congr., 3rd sess. (Washington, D.C.: U.S. Government Printing Office, 1911).

18. This conclusion was arrived at by reviewing the data of immigrants debarred for trachoma as compiled by the USPHS, 1897–1924. See *Annual Reports of the Supervising Surgeon General of the USMHS/USPHS,* 1897–1925. See also Memorandum from Victor Safford to the Surgeon General, June 14, 1911, box 5, Papers of the Immigration Restriction League, Houghton Library, Harvard University. For a synthesis of the statistics of immigration and health in the United States during the great wave of immigration, see Amy L. Fairchild, *Science at the Borders: Immigrant Medical Inspection and the Shaping of the Modern Industrial Labor Force* (Baltimore: Johns Hopkins University Press, 2003).

19. James Jones, *Bad Blood: The Tuskegee Syphilis Experiment* (New York: Free Press, 1993), pp. 54, 113–32.

20. T. Clark and J. W. Schereschewsky, *Trachoma: Its Character and Effects* (Washington, D.C.: U.S. Government Printing Office, 1907), p. 12.

21. John McMullan, "Trachoma: Its Prevalence and Control Among Immigrants," *Journal of the American Medical Association* 61 (1913): 1110–13. Interestingly, the running title for this article was "Keep Trachoma Out."

22. *Reports of the Immigration Commission,* vol. 4, pp. 93–124.

23. Irving Howe, *World of Our Fathers: The Journey of the East European Jews to America and the Life They Found and Made* (New York: Harcourt Brace Jovanovich, 1976), p. 5. See also Howard Markel, *Quarantine!: East European Jewish Immigrants and the New York City Epidemics of 1892* (Baltimore: Johns Hopkins University Press, 1997), pp. 16–21.

24. Julius Boldt, *Trachoma,* trans. J. H. Parsons and T. Snowball, with an introduction by E. Treacher Collins (London: Hodder and Stoughton, 1904), pp. 42–43, 50. (Originally published as *Das Trachom als Volks—und Heereskrankheit* [Berlin:

Hirschwald, 1903].) See also G. E. de Schweinitz, "Trachoma and Common Forms of Conjunctivitis," in *Military Ophthalmic Surgery*, ed. A. Greenwood (Philadelphia: Lea and Febiger, 1917), p. 64.

25. Allen Busby, "Trachoma," *Long Island Medical Journal* 1 (1907): 373–75.

26. See *Evteiskii Medtsinski Golos* 2–3 (1908): M. Mandlestamm, "Trachoma and Emigration to America," 90–96; G. M. Rabinovich, "Emigrants and Trachoma," 97–105; L. M. Rosenfeld, "Trachoma and Jewish Emigration," 106–17; "Questionnaire About Trachoma, Favus and Herpes Tonsurans," 119–23. I am indebted to Dr. Lisa Epstein of the YIVO Institute for pointing these articles out to me and to Natasha Rekhter of the University of Michigan for translating these articles from Russian to English.

27. Mandlestamm, "Trachoma and Emigration to America," p. 90.

28. Boldt, *Trachoma*, pp. 42–43, 50.

29. Minutes of the National Jewish Immigration Committee, Dec. 1, 1912, Collections of the American Jewish Historical Society, Waltham, Mass. The National Jewish Immigration Committee met regularly throughout the first three decades of the twentieth century in active support of these and similar causes.

30. The American Jewish Committee also met regularly to discuss immigration issues. The committee and its proceedings have been formally preserved during this period in the *American Jewish Yearbook* (Philadelphia: Jewish Publication Society, 1900–1924).

31. Cecilia Razovsky, *What Every Emigrant Should Know: A Simple Pamphlet for the Guidance and Benefit of Prospective Immigrants to the United States,* Yiddish and English eds. (New York: National Council of Jewish Women, Department of Immigrant Aid, 1922), pp. 1, 18.

32. Trachoma poster, Fund for the Relief of Jewish Victims of the War in Eastern Europe and the Federation of Ukrainian Jews, London, 1923, YIVO Institute for Jewish Studies, New York City.

33. Lisa Epstein, "Caring for the Soul's House: The Jews of Russia and Health Care, 1860–1914" (Ph.D. diss., Yale University, 1995); Nancy Frieden, *Russian Physicians in an Era of Reform and Revolution, 1856–1905* (Princeton: Princeton University Press, 1981); Susan Solomon and John F. Hutchinson, eds., *Health and Society in Revolutionary Russia* (Bloomington: Indiana University Press, 1990).

34. Rosenfeld, "Trachoma and Jewish Emigration."

35. Examination techniques are summarized in Charles May, *Manual of the Diseases of the Eye* (Baltimore: Williams & Wilkins, 1968), pp. 97–100; Casey Wood, ed., *The American Encyclopedia and Dictionary of Ophthalmology*, vol. 17 (Chicago: Cleveland Press, 1913–21), pp. 12878–944; U.S. Treasury Department, *Book of Instructions for the Medical Inspection of Immigrants* (Washington D.C.: U.S. Government Printing Office, 1903); U.S. Treasury Office, *Regulations Governing the Medical Inspection of Aliens, August 1917* (Washington, D.C.: U.S. Government Printing Office, 1917). For the types of instruments used to evert the eyelids (other than the fingers and a buttonhook), see Charles Truax, *The Mechanics of Surgery Comprising Detailed Descriptions, Illustrations, and Lists of the Instruments, Appliances and Furniture Necessary in Modern Surgical Art* (Chicago:

W. B. Conkey, 1899), Collections of the Center for the History of Medicine, University of Michigan, Ann Arbor.

36. Maurice Fishberg, "Report to the Commissioner-General of Immigration, Frank P. Sargent," in *Annual Report of the Commissioner General of Immigration to the Secretary of Commerce and Labor for 1905* (Washington, D.C.: U.S. Government Printing Office, 1905), pp. 50–56.

37. For a description of the American responses to the 1892 cholera epidemic, see Markel, *Quarantine!*. For a magisterial description of the 1892 epidemic in Germany and throughout Europe, see Richard Evans, *Death in Hamburg: Society and Politics in the Cholera Years, 1830–1910* (Oxford, Eng.: Clarendon, 1987).

38. Fishberg, "Report," pp. 52–53. See also Lamar Cecil, *Albert Ballin: Business and Politics in Imperial Germany, 1888–1918* (Princeton: Princeton University Press, 1967), pp. 24, 40–43.

39. Benjamin Croft, "Trachoma," *Boston Medical and Surgical Journal* 155 (1906): 305–7. For other contemporary accounts that cast suspicion both on the medical inspection process and the validity of the diagnoses themselves, see A. L. Benedict, "Trachoma and Immigration," *New York Medical Journal* 78 (1903): 373–74; Ellice Alger, "The Epidemic of So-Called Trachoma," *New York Medical Journal* 80 (1904): 684–87; Howard Hansell, "Trachoma, Clinically and Socially Considered," *New York Medical Journal* 85 (1907): 486–88.

40. Fishberg, "Report," p. 54.

41. Ibid., p. 56; Edward Steiner, *From Alien to Citizen* (New York: Revell, 1914), p. 31; *Der Tog* (The New York Yiddish Day), Dec. 14, 1908, p. 2. The term *shlepp* literally means "to drag" but was used in this case for the term "runner," or one who promised to "run" immigrants across the border without hindrance from the immigration authorities.

42. The INS Special Boards of Inquiry case collections are, unfortunately, replete with such tragic cases. See INS Collection 60A/600, RG 85, National Archives Records Administration. The separation of families, of course, was not restricted to East European Jews; one finds similar tragedies among the other major immigrant groups during this period as well.

43. Goldenbaum File, HIAS Collection, Ellis Island Bureau, YIVO Institute.

44. A. F. MacCallan, *Trachoma and Its Complications in Egypt* (Cambridge, Eng.: Cambridge University Press, 1913), p. 3. See also *Report of the Trachoma Conference in the Jewish Colony of Palestine of 1914* (Jerusalem: The Jewish Health Bureau, 1915, in Hebrew); Joseph Krimsky, "Trachoma in Palestine," *Long Island Medical Journal* 14, no. 4 (1920): 171–76.

45. Mary Karasch, "Ophthalmia (Conjunctivitis and Trachoma)," in *The Cambridge World History of Human Disease,* ed. Kenneth Kiple (New York: Cambridge University Press, 1993), pp. 897–906.

46. See *Reports of the Immigration Commission, Conditions in Europe,* vol. 4, pp. 93–124; *Annual Report of the Commissioner General of Immigration, 1905,* pp. 50–56; *Annual Report of the Supervising Surgeon General of the U.S. Marine Hospital Service, 1900,* p. 523; Allan McLaughlin, "Italian and Other Latin Immigrants," *Popular Science Monthly* 65 (1904): 341–49.

47. Howe, *World of Our Fathers*, pp. 39–42; Gerald Sorin, *A Time for Building: The Third Migration, 1880–1920* (Baltimore: Johns Hopkins University Press, 1992), pp. 45–47; Cecil, *Ballin*, pp. 7–14, 38–39.

48. John Malcolm Brinnin, *The Sway of the Grand Saloon* (London: Arlington, 1986), pp. 164, 261–62.

49. Reed, "Immigration and the Public Health," pp. 320–28. Quote is from p. 323.

50. E. W. Smith, *Passenger Ships of the World: Past and Present* (Boston: Dean, 1963), pp. 236–37; *Morton Allan Directory of European Passenger Steamship Arrivals for the Years 1890 to 1930 at the Port of New York* (Baltimore: Genealogical Publishing, 1980), p. 190.

51. Howe, *World of Our Fathers*, pp. 39–42; *Reports of the U.S. Immigration Commission, 1907–1910*, vol. 39: *Immigration Legislation: Steerage Legislation, 1819–1908*, U.S. Senate Document #758, 61st Congr., 3rd sess. (Washington, D.C.: U.S. Government Printing Office, 1911), pp. 335–485.

52. Ship's manifest, *S.S. San Guglielmo*, Sept. 23, 1916.

53. Frederick Taylor, *The Principles of Scientific Management* (New York: Harper & Brothers, 1911).

54. *Baltimore News-American*, Sept. 2, 1892, p. 6.

55. These numbers are drawn from Kraut, *Silent Travelers*, p. 61.

56. Victor Safford, *Immigration Problems: Personal Experiences of an Official* (New York: Dodd, Mead, 1925), pp. 244–57. Quote is from pp. 244–45.

57. For positive accounts of the medical inspection process, see Reed, "Going Through Ellis Island" and "Immigration and the Public Health"; McLaughlin, "How Immigrants Are Inspected"; Henry, "Among the Immigrants."

58. See, for example, the testimony of the British ambassador to the United States, A. C. Geddes, on a visit to Ellis Island in 1923, where he describes a physician doing serial inguinal-genital hernia examinations on young men without washing hands in between patients. *Dispatch from Her Majesty's Ambassador at Washington Reporting on Conditions at Ellis Island Immigration Station*, London, 1923.

59. Theodore Roosevelt to V. H. Metcalf, Feb. 22, 1906, in *The Letters of Theodore Roosevelt*, vol. 5, ed. Elting Morison (Cambridge: Harvard University Press, 1952), pp. 162–63.

60. Disinfectant regulations are clearly codified by 1917; see USPHS, *Regulations Governing the Medical Inspection of Aliens, August, 1917*, Miscellaneous Publication No. 5 (Washington, D.C.: U.S. Government Printing Office, 1917), p. 19. Most of the extant photographs in the National Archives and Library of Congress collections were taken between 1915 and 1924. Many are easily surmised to be staged photographs with careful posing of the immigrants and the inspectors. The overwhelming majority of these photographs (82 percent), however, also reveal a paucity of sanitary measures, such as an easy means of hand washing. This prompts the question, if the photographs were posed and sanitary technique was standard operational procedure as listed in the USPHS regulations, why did not all of the photographs have a staged portable sink or basin?

61. See, for example, E. H. Mullan photograph circa 1924 inspecting Chinese immi-

grants for trachoma using his thumb and forefingers, National Library of Medicine Collections, Bethesda, Md. (#AD18050).

62. Data compiled from *Annual Reports of the U.S. Commissioner General of Immigration, 1900–1920.*

63. Louis Frank to Samuel Littman, Apr. 24, 1915, HIAS Ellis Island Bureau Cases (Miscellaneous Sick Cases), HIAS Collections, YIVO Institute, New York. This letter is typical of much of the correspondence between HIAS and the local hospitals with regard to accepting trachoma cases, which were well known to be chronic and expensive to treat.

64. See "Annual Reports of the Commissioner of Ellis Island, 1902–1909, 1909–1913," William Williams Papers, box 5, Rare Book and Manuscript Collections, New York Public Library, New York City.

65. Ronald Sanders, *The Downtown Jews: Portraits of an Immigrant Generation* (New York: Harper & Row, 1969); Moses Rischin, *The Promised City: New York's Jews, 1870–1914* (Cambridge: Harvard University Press, 1962); *The Jewish Communal Register of New York City, 1917–1918*, 2nd ed. (New York: Jewish Community of New York City, 1918); Arthur Goren, *New York Jews and the Quest for Community: The Kehillah Experiment, 1908–1922* (New York: Columbia University Press, 1970).

66. There did exist earlier organizations such as the Hebrew Sheltering and Immigrant Aid Society, which joined forces with HIAS in 1909, and the Hebrew Emigrant Aid Society, which had two incarnations in the late 1870s and early 1880s. The major difference between all of these organizations when compared to HIAS was that HIAS was founded and operated by East European Jews (as opposed to German Jews) who looked on their clients as brothers rather than objects of charity. See Mark Wischnitzer, *Visas to Freedom: The History of HIAS* (Cleveland and New York: World, 1956).

67. Tina Levitan, *Islands of Compassion: A History of the Jewish Hospitals of New York* (New York: Twayne, 1964); David Rosner, *A Once Charitable Enterprise: Hospitals and Health Care in Brooklyn and New York, 1885–1915* (Cambridge, Eng.: Cambridge University Press, 1982).

68. See, for example, the Aron Genbarg File, HIAS Ellis Island Bureau, MKM 10.8, files 37–42, HIAS Collections, YIVO Institute, New York City. Genbarg was sent back to Russia because his family could not raise the funds despite frequent requests from HIAS agents.

69. Ibid. The definition "social group" does not do justice to the Yiddish term *landsmanshaftn;* more broadly, they were immigrant benevolent societies whose members shared strong geographical, social, and cultural ties to their East European *shtetls.* Michael Weisser, *A Brotherhood of Memory: Jewish Landsmanshaftn in the New World* (New York: Basic Books, 1985), p. 4. See also Daniel Soyer, *Jewish Immigrant Associations and American Identity in New York, 1880–1939* (Cambridge: Harvard University Press, 1997); Molly Picon and Jean Grillo, *Molly!: An Autobiography* (New York: Simon & Schuster, 1980), p. 46.

70. For example, the first full-length Yiddish drama on an American subject, *Die Emi-*

*gratsie kein Amerika* (Emigration to America), was written and produced by Joseph Lateiner in New York in 1886. The use of the immigration experience as a source for dramatic inspiration only increased over the next three decades as East European immigration reached its peak. Some of the best-known productions of this genre included Allen Shomer's 1911 play, *At Sea and Ellis Island,* Jacob Adler's 1913 production of *The Immigrant,* and Jacob Gordin's 1914 productions, *The Russian Jew in America* and *Dementia Americana.* Some of the most popular Yiddish songs about the immigration experience include "Shikt a Tiket" (Send a Ticket), "Frayhayt Statue" (Statue of Liberty), "Kesl Gardn" (Castle Garden), and "Elis Ayland" (Ellis Island). Jacob Adler, *A Life on the Stage: A Memoir,* trans. and ed. Lulla Adler Rosenfeld (New York: Knopf, 1999); Lulla Adler Rosenfeld, *The Yiddish Theatre and Jacob P. Adler* (New York: Shapolsky, 1988); Nahma Sandrow, *Vagabond Stars: A World History of Yiddish Theater* (New York: Limelight, 1986); David Lifson, *The Yiddish Theatre in America* (New York: Yoseloff, 1965); Jerry Silverman, *The Yiddish Song Book* (New York: Stein & Day, 1983), pp. 152–53, 155–57, 161.

71. Goldenbaum File, HIAS Collection, Ellis Island Bureau, YIVO Institute. The Yiddish word *noodge* might be translated as "the frequent needling, bothering, and advocating for a specific cause or goal."

72. Goldenbaum's treatment regimen is extracted from his HIAS case file, reel # MK 10.8, YIVO Institute; T. Clark and J. W. Schereschewsky, *Trachoma: Its Character and Effects* (Washington, D.C.: U.S. Government Printing Office, 1907), pp. 30–32.

73. Sholom Aleichem, the pen name of Sholom Rabinowitz, was the most popular and beloved of Yiddish writers, both in Eastern Europe and the New World. The "Off for America" stories were translated by Marian Weinstein of the New York Yiddish daily newspaper, *Der Tog* (The Day), where they were originally published in Yiddish under the supervision of Sholom Aleichem, in *The New York World Magazine* beginning Jan. 2, 1916, and then, serially, in the following issues: Jan. 9, pp. 13, 17; Jan. 16, p. 13; Jan. 23, p. 12; Jan. 30, p. 12; Feb. 13, p. 13; Feb. 27, p. 13. The last few installments were published posthumously (the writer died in New York City on May 14), and the novel's last, unfinished chapter represents the author's final written words. The next day, he was buried in Brooklyn after what was then considered one of the largest funeral processions ever held in New York City. For a memoir of this exciting conclusion to Sholom Aleichem's writing career, see Marie Waife-Goldberg, *My Father, Sholom Aleichem* (New York: Schocken, 1968), pp. 302–5; and Ellen D. Kellman, "Sholom Aleichem's Funeral (New York 1916): The Making of a National Pageant," *YIVO Annual* 20 (1991): 277–304.

74. Sholom Aleichem, "Off for the Golden Land," *Jewish Immigration Bulletin* 7, no. 1 (February 1917): 10–11. Quote is from p. 10. This is a better translation of the March 26, 1916, installment that appeared in the *New York World Magazine.*

75. Goldenbaum File, HIAS Collection, YIVO Institute.

76. Ibid., De Sola Pool to HIAS, Jan. 22, 1917. See also *The Jewish Communal Register of New York City, 1917–1918* (New York: Kehillah-Jewish Community of New York, 1918), p. 1401.

77. Goldenbaum File, Jan. 29, 1916; Doris Goldstein, *From Generation to Generation:*

*A Centennial History of Congregation Ahavath Achim, 1887–1987* (Atlanta: Capricorn, 1987); Steven Hertzberg, *Strangers Within the Gate City: The Jews of Atlanta, 1845–1915* (Philadelphia: Jewish Publication Society, 1978).

78. Leonard Dinnerstein, *The Leo Frank Case* (New York: Columbia University Press, 1968); Nancy MacLean, "The Leo Frank Case Reconsidered," *Journal of American History* 78 (December 1991): 917–48.

79. *Atlanta Constitution*, Apr. 8, 1917, 1:3.

80. *Annual Report for 2001: International Trachoma Initiative* (New York: International Trachoma Initiative, 2001).

81. Ibid.; Howard Markel, "Germ Warfare," *New York Times*, Sept. 6, 2003, p. A23.

82. Rudolf Virchow, "Report on the Typhus Epidemic in Upper Silesia," in *Collected Essays on Public Health and Epidemiology*, vol. 1, ed. L. J. Rather (Canton, Mass.: Science History Publications, 1985), p. 213.

83. Book of Proverbs 29:18.


CHAPTER FOUR • LICE, TYPHUS, AND RIOTS ON THE TEXAS-MEXICO BORDER

1. *El Paso Times*, Jan. 29, 1917, p. 1.

2. Ibid.; *El Paso Herald*, Jan. 29, 1917, p. 1; *New York Times*, Jan. 29, 1917, p. 6.

3. Victoria Harden, "Typhus, Epidemic," in *The Cambridge World History of Human Disease*, ed. Kenneth Kiple (New York: Cambridge University Press, 1993), pp. 1080–84; S. B. Wolbach, J. L. Todd, and F. W. Palfrey, *The Etiology and Pathology of Typhus* (Cambridge: League of Red Cross Societies at the Harvard University Press, 1922); Thomas McCrae, "Typhus Fever," in *Modern Medicine: Its Theory and Practice*, vol. 2, ed. William Osler (Philadelphia: Lea and Febiger, 1907), pp. 231–44.

4. Charles Murchison, *A Treatise on the Continued Fevers of Great Britain* (London: Longmans, Green, 1884), pp. 121–22.

5. Hans Zinsser, *Rats, Lice and History* (Boston: Atlantic Monthly Press/Little, Brown, 1935), pp. 254–62; John Anderson and Joseph Goldberger, "The Etiology of *Tabardillo* or Mexican Typhus: An Experimental Investigation," *Journal of Medical Research* 22 (1910): 469–81.

6. George Rosen, "Tenements and Typhus in New York City, 1840–1875," *American Journal of Public Health* 62 (1972): 590–93.

7. Jacob Riis, *How the Other Half Lives: Studies Among the Tenements of New York* (New York: Scribner's, 1890), p. 109; Howard Markel, *Quarantine!: East European Jewish Immigrants and the New York City Epidemics of 1892* (Baltimore: Johns Hopkins University Press, 1997).

8. Kimberly Pelis, "Pasteur's Imperial Missionary: Charles Nicolle (1866–1936) and the Pasteur Institute of Tunis" (Ph.D. diss., Johns Hopkins University, 1995); Victoria Harden, *Rocky Mountain Spotted Fever: History of a Twentieth-Century Disease* (Baltimore: Johns Hopkins University Press, 1990), pp. 69–71; E. H. Ackerknecht, *History and Geography of the Most Important Diseases* (New York: Hafner, 1965), pp. 32–43; L. Gross, "How Charles Nicolle of the Pasteur Institute Discovered That Epidemic Typhus Is Transmitted by Lice: Reminiscences from

My Years at the Pasteur Institute in Paris," *Proceedings of the National Academy of Sciences* 93, no. 20 (1996): 10539–40. There are other variants of typhus that were at one time considered "different" diseases but subsequently shown to be the same infection, including Brill's disease and *el tabardillo.*

9. See, for example, T. Philip Terry, *Terry's Mexico: A New Guidebook to the Mexican Republic,* 2nd ed. (Boston: Houghton Mifflin, 1909), p. xxviii.

10. Francis Redewell, "Typhus Fever," *Southwestern Medicine* 1 (1917): 31–39. Quote is from p. 39.

11. Zinsser, *Rats, Lice and History,* p. 178.

12. Ibid., pp. 221–23.

13. Walter Lippmann, "Legendary John Reed," *The New Republic* Dec. 12, 1914, pp. 15–16. For a superb biography of Lippmann, see Ronald Steel, *Walter Lippmann and the American Century* (New York: Vintage, 1981).

14. John Reed, *Insurgent Mexico* (New York: Appleton, 1914), p. 1.

15. Ibid., pp. 3–4.

16. *El Paso Herald,* Mar. 7–8, 1914, p. 8.

17. Much of this section is drawn from Mario García, *Desert Immigrants: The Mexicans of El Paso, 1880–1920* (New Haven: Yale University Press, 1981). See also Samuel Bryan, "Mexican Immigrants in the United States," *Survey* 28 (1912): 726–30; Victor Clark, "Mexican Labor in the United States," U.S. Department of Commerce and Labor, *Bureau of Labor Bulletin* 78 (1908; reprint, *Mexican Labor in the U.S.,* ed. C. E. Cortes et al. [New York: Arno, 1974]).

18. John Reed, "El Paso," unpublished manuscript (bMS AM 1091, #1147), Reed Papers, Houghton Library, Harvard University.

19. García, *Desert Immigrants,* pp. 1–8.

20. Mark Reisler, *By the Sweat of Their Brow: Mexican Immigrant Labor in the United States, 1900–1940* (Westport, Ct.: Greenwood, 1976); Howard Markel and Alexandra Stern, "Which Face, Whose Nation?: Immigration, Public Health, and the Construction of Disease at America's Ports and Borders," in *Immigration Research for a New Century: Multidisciplinary Perspectives,* ed. N. Foner, R. G. Rumbaut, and S. J. Gold (New York: Russell Sage Foundation, 2000), pp. 93–112.

21. Reisler, *By the Sweat of Their Brow,* pp. 24–48.

22. García, *Desert Immigrants,* pp. 6, 127–54.

23. *El Paso Times,* June 17, 1910, p. 8.

24. Both quotes cited in Eddie Lou Miller, "The History of Private Welfare Agencies in El Paso, 1866–1930" (master's thesis, University of Texas at El Paso, 1969), pp. 72–73.

25. Quoted in *El Paso Herald,* Feb. 9, 1915, p. 4.

26. *El Paso Times,* Jan. 27, 1903, p. 1.

27. *Seraphic Report Regarding Conditions on the Mexican Border, 1906–1907,* case file 51423/1, reel 1, RG 85, microfilm records of the INS, series A, part 2, Mexican Immigration, 1906–1930 (Bethesda, Md.: American University Publications).

28. *Annual Reports of the Surgeon General of the U.S. Public Health Service, 1900–1930* (Washington, D.C.: U.S. Government Printing Office, 1900–1930).

29. Carlos Husk, "Typhus Fever," *Bulletin of the El Paso County Medical Society* 78 (1916): 75–79 (quote is from p. 78). For a brief description of Husk, see Friedrich

Katz, *The Life and Times of Pancho Villa* (Stanford: Stanford University Press, 1998), p. 6.

30. *El Paso Herald,* Feb. 21, 1916, p. 1; *Survey,* Mar. 4, 1916, p. 652.

31. *El Paso Herald,* Mar. 10, 1916, p. 13; Mar. 11–12, 1916, p. 1; "Quarantine," *Bulletin of the El Paso County Medical Society* 8 (1916): 136–37; C. C. Pierce, "Typhus Fever," *Bulletin of the El Paso County Medical Society* 8 (1916): 173–76, 256–57; *El Paso Herald,* Apr. 6, 1916, p. 12.

32. J. W. Tappan to U.S. Surgeon General Rupert Blue, Mar. 1, 1916, El Paso Quarantine Station, 1904–24, RG 90, USPHS, file 1248, National Archives Records Administration, College Park, Md.

33. For an obituary and description of Buttner's illness, as well as plans to raise money for his surviving family, see *El Paso Morning Times,* Mar. 8, 1916, p. 8; C. C. Pierce, "Cases of Typhus Fever in the City of El Paso, January 1–June 30, 1916," file 2126, RG 90, box 207, file 1, USPHS, National Archives Records Administration.

34. *El Paso Herald,* Mar. 6, 7, 8, 1916, p. 1; *El Paso Morning Times,* Mar. 8, 1916, p. 1.

35. *San Antonio Express,* Mar. 9, 1916, p. 1.

36. Ibid.

37. *El Paso Herald,* Mar. 8, 1916, p. 1; *El Paso Morning Times,* Mar. 8, 1916, p. 1.

38. Mario Acevedo, interview by Oscar J. Martínez, tape recording #153B, May 1, 1975, University of Texas at El Paso, Institute of Oral History, pp. 21–22. Other accounts of Villa's revenge can be found in the account of Brigadier General S.L.A. Marshall, interview by Richard Estrada, tape recording #181, July 5, 7, 9, 11, 19, 1975, University of Texas at El Paso, Institute of Oral History; Tom Mahoney, "The Columbus Raid," *Southwest Review* 17 (1932): 164. See also Alexandra Stern, "Buildings, Boundaries, and Blood: Medicalization and Nation-Building on the U.S.-Mexico Border, 1910–1930," *Hispanic American Historical Review* 79 (1999): 41–81; Katz, *Life and Times of Pancho Villa,* pp. 545–82.

39. J. W. Tappan to Surgeon General Rupert Blue, June 23, 1916, El Paso Quarantine Station, 1904–1924, RG 90, USPHS, file 1248, National Archives Records Administration.

40. B. J. Lloyd to Surgeon General Blue, June 27, 1916, RG 90, USPHS, file 1248, National Archives Records Administration.

41. Ibid., July 5, 1916.

42. Charles Montague to U.S. Secretary of State, forwarded to USPHS Quarantine Station at El Paso, Aug. 30, 1916, RG 90, USPHS, file 1248, National Archives Records Administration.

43. Ibid.

44. Friedrich Katz, *The Secret War in Mexico: Europe, the United States and the Mexican Revolution* (Chicago: University of Chicago Press, 1981).

45. *New York Times,* Aug. 13, 1916, p. 5.

46. *El Paso Herald,* Jan. 1–2, 1917, p. 2; Jan. 4, 1917, p. 2; *El Paso Morning Times,* Jan. 5, 1917, p. 1; *El Paso Herald,* Jan. 5, 1917, p. 2.

47. *El Paso Morning Times,* Jan. 5, 1917, p. 1.

48. Correspondence between C. C. Pierce and Surgeon General Blue, Jan. 1–25, 1917, RG 90, USPHS, file 126, National Archives Records Administration.

49. C. C. Pierce to all Quarantine Officers, Collectors of Customs, U.S. Immigration Officials and others along the Mexican Border (circular), Jan. 23, 1917, RG 90, USPHS, file 126, National Archives Records Administration. The Mexican Punitive Expedition officially concluded on February 5, 1917, when the last American troops left Mexican soil.

50. *El Paso Morning Times,* Jan. 28, 1917, p. 1.

51. *El Paso Times,* Jan. 29, 1917, p. 1; *El Paso Herald,* Jan. 29, 1917, p. 1; *New York Times,* Jan. 29, 1917, p. 6.

52. This dynamic is discussed in an article by Eric Schmitt, "Trapped: Americans (a) Love (b) Hate Immigrants," *New York Times,* Jan. 14, 2001, sec. 4, p. 1.

53. *El Paso Times,* Jan. 29, 1917, p. 1.

54. *New York Times,* Jan. 29, 1917, p. 6; *El Paso Times,* Jan. 29, 1917, p. 1; *El Paso Herald,* Jan. 29, 1917, p. 1; *El Paso Times,* Jan. 30, 1917, p. 1; *San Antonio Express,* Jan. 29, 1917, p. 1.

55. "Excitative to the Patriotic People of Juárez from the Mayor, Melchor Herrera," Jan. 29, 1917, El Paso Quarantine Station, RG 90, USPHS, file 126, National Archives Records Administration.

56. Felix López Urdiales, interview by Oscar J. Martínez, tape recording #144C, Feb. 22, 1974, University of Texas at El Paso, Institute of Oral History, pp. 5–6.

57. C. C. Pierce to Surgeon General Blue, Feb. 6, 1917, El Paso Quarantine Station, RG 90, USPHS, file 126, National Archives Records Administration. Similar letters complaining about the Mexican threat of disease and the uncooperative nature of the Mexican health officials are also in this file beginning in late January and continuing throughout the calendar year of 1917.

58. *Public Health Reports,* June 1, 1917, p. 865, and June 29, 1917, p. 1057; Report from C. C. Pierce to Surgeon General Blue, Jan. 9, 1917, RG 90 Central File 1897–1923, file 1248, National Archives Records Administration; Stern, "Buildings, Boundaries, and Blood."

59. *El Paso Herald,* Feb. 26, 1917, p. 4. For examples of requests to the U.S. surgeon general to lift the quarantine regulations along the border, see letter from Andres García, inspector general of consulaters of Mexico, to Surgeon General Blue, July 20, 1917, and letter from G. C. Carruthers, on behalf of the Mayor of Juárez, to Secretary of State Robert Lansing, Aug. 30, 1917; for examples of letters denying such requests, see letter from Z. J. Cobb to Surgeon J. W. Tappan, July 23, 1917, and Surgeon J. W. Tappan to Surgeon General Blue, Sept. 21, 1917, El Paso Quarantine Station, RG 90, USPHS, file 126, National Archives Records Administration.

60. James J. Davis, "Memorandum for the Commissioner General of Immigration," Feb. 29, 1924, National Archives, INS, RG 85, series A, part 2 (microfilm 52903/29).

61. Vera Sturges, "Mexican Immigrants," *The Survey Graphic,* July 2, 1921, pp. 470–71.

62. Robert Rosenstone, *Romantic Revolutionary: A Biography of John Reed* (New York: Knopf, 1975), pp. 379–82.

63. Paul Weindling, *Epidemics and Genocide in Eastern Europe, 1890–1945* (Oxford, Eng.: Oxford University Press, 2000); Wolbach, Todd, and Palfrey, *Etiology and*

*Pathology of Typhus;* Charles Roland, *Courage Under Siege: Starvation, Disease and Death in the Warsaw Ghetto* (New York: Oxford University Press, 1992).

64. John Tappan, "Protective Health Measures on the United States–Mexico Border," *Journal of the American Medical Association* 87, no. 13 (1926): 1022–26.

65. For a superb analysis of this process of demarcation, see Stern, "Buildings, Boundaries, and Blood."

66. See George Sánchez, *Becoming Mexican American: Ethnicity, Culture and Identity in Chicano Los Angeles, 1900–1945* (New York: Oxford University Press, 1993), pp. 38–62. For an excellent description of how the border was "solidified," see also Report of Mounted Guards Heston B. Martin and Alvis C. Taylor, 1923, file 1169, Laredo and San Antonio, Texas, RG 90, USPHS, Central File 1897–1923, National Archives Records Administration.

67. Adam Clymer, "Bush and Texas Have Not Set High Priority on Health Care," *New York Times,* Apr. 11, 2000, p. A1.

68. Hippocrates, *Epidemics,* book 1, part 11, in *Hippocrates,* vol. 1, *Ancient Medicine. Airs, Waters, Places. Epidemics 1 & 3. The Oath. Precepts. Nutriment,* trans. W. H. S. Jones (Cambridge: Harvard University Press, 1923), p. 165.


CHAPTER FIVE • NO ONE'S IDEA OF A TROPICAL PARADISE:
HAITIAN IMMIGRANTS AND AIDS

1. Anne-Christine D'Adesky, "Silence + Death = AIDS in Haiti," *The Advocate,* May 21, 1991, pp. 30–36. Quote is from p. 31.

2. "Medical Inspection of Immigrants (AIDS)," *Federal Register,* Apr. 23, 1986: 15354–55; "Medical Inspection of Immigrants," *Federal Register,* June 8, 1987: 21607–608; Howard Markel, "A U.S. Agency Shuts the Gates on AIDS Victims," *Baltimore Evening Sun,* June 6, 1990, p. A13; Laurie Garrett, "Health Threat or Scapegoat?: Travelers with HIV Are Caught in a Political Storm," *Newsday,* Aug. 4, 1991, p. 51; A. L. Fairchild and E. A. Tynan, "Policies of Containment: Immigration in the Era of AIDS," *American Journal of Public Health* 84 (1994): 2011–22; L. O. Gostin et al., "Screening Immigrants and International Travelers for the Human Immunodeficiency Virus," *New England Journal of Medicine* 322 (1990): 1743–46.

3. Mark Danner, "Beyond the Mountains," *The New Yorker,* part 1, Nov. 27, 1989, pp. 55–100; part 2, Dec. 4, 1989, pp. 68–141; part 3, Dec. 11, 1989, pp. 100–131. Columbus story is from Part 2, p. 77. Others have attributed this story to Napoleon in 1807.

4. Michel Laguerre, *American Odyssey: Haitians in New York City* (Ithaca: Cornell University Press, 1984); Anthony Catanese, *Haitians: Migration and Diaspora* (Boulder, Colo.: Westview, 1999).

5. Robert Heinl, Jr., and Nancy Heinl, *Written in Blood: The Story of the Haitian People, 1492–1995,* rev. by Michael Heinl (Lanham, Md.: University Press of America, 1996).

6. Paul Farmer, "The Power of the Poor in Haiti," *America* 164 (Mar. 9, 1991):

260–67; T. D. Allman, "After Baby Doc," *Vanity Fair* 52, no. 1 (1989): 74–116; Tracy Kidder, *Mountains Beyond Mountains: The Quest of Dr. Paul Farmer, A Man Who Would Cure the World* (New York: Random House, 2003).

7. For an exploration of this relationship, see Matthew Frye Jacobson, *Whiteness of a Different Color: European Immigrants and the Alchemy of Race* (Cambridge: Harvard University Press, 1998); Leon Pamphile, *Haitians and African Americans: A Heritage of Tragedy and Hope* (Gainesville: University Press of Florida, 2001).

8. The historian Edgar La Selve is quoted in Heinl and Heinl, *Written in Blood,* p. 9. See also C. L. R. James, *The Black Jacobins: Toussaint L'Ouverture and the San Domingo Revolution,* rev. ed. (New York: Vintage, 1963); Walter LaFeber, *The New Empire: An Interpretation of American Expansion, 1860–1898,* 35th Anniversary ed. (Ithaca: Cornell University Press, 1998). France finally granted Haiti its "official Independence" on April 17, 1825.

9. Heinl and Heinl, *Written in Blood,* pp. 560–635.

10. Quoted in ibid., pp. 571–72.

11. Ibid., pp. 100–101.

12. Danner, "Beyond the Mountains," part 2, pp. 125–29, 131.

13. Heinl and Heinl, *Written in Blood,* p. 634; Michel-Rolph Trouillot, *Haiti, State Against Nation: The Origins and Legacy of Duvalierism* (New York: Monthly Review Press, 1990), p. 200; Paul Farmer, *AIDS and Accusation: Haiti and the Geography of Blame* (Berkeley: University of California Press, 1992), pp. 143–48.

14. *Spartacus International Gay Guide* (Amsterdam: Spartacus, 1981), p. 6.

15. See, for example, Edward Hooper, *The River: A Journey to the Source of HIV and AIDS* (Boston: Little, Brown, 1999); Randy Shilts, *And the Band Played On: Politics, People and the AIDS Epidemic* (New York: St. Martin's, 1987); Luc Montagnier, *Virus: The Co-Discoverer of HIV Tracks Its Rampage and Charts the Future,* trans. Stephen Sartarelli (New York: Norton, 2000); Donald G. McNeil, "Researchers Have New Theory on Origin of AIDS Virus," *New York Times,* June 13, 2003, p. A25.

16. Quoted in Claude Quétel, *History of Syphilis,* trans. Judith Braddock and Brian Pike (Baltimore: Johns Hopkins University Press, 1990), p. 37.

17. Ibid., pp. 31–49; Ralph H. Major, ed., *Classic Descriptions of Disease,* 3rd ed. (Springfield, Ill.: Thomas, 1945), pp. 12–51.

18. Mirko Grmek, *History of AIDS: Emergence and Origin of a Modern Pandemic* (Princeton: Princeton University Press, 1990), pp. 158–61, 168–70. For a broader discussion of such phenomena, see W. H. McNeill, *Plagues and Peoples* (Garden City, N.Y.: Anchor/Doubleday, 1976).

19. Quoted in Grmek, *History of AIDS,* p. 170.

20. Warren Johnson and Jean Pape, "AIDS in Haiti," in *AIDS Pathogenesis and Treatment,* ed. Jay Levy (New York: Dekker, 1989), pp. 65–78. See also J. Pape and W. Johnson, "Epidemiology of AIDS in the Caribbean," in *Baillière's Clinical Tropical Medicine and Communicable Diseases* 3, no. 1 (1988): 31–42.

21. S. O. Murray, "A Note on Haitian Tolerance of Homosexuality," in *Male Homosexuality in Central and South America,* ed. S. Murray (New York: Gay Academic Union, 1987), pp. 92–100.

22. William Osler, "Internal Medicine as a Vocation," in *Aequanimitas with Other Addresses*, 3rd ed. (Philadelphia: Blakiston, 1932), pp. 133–45. Quote is from p. 134. For biographical information on Osler, see Harvey Cushing, *The Life of Sir William Osler* (Oxford, Eng.: Clarendon Press of Oxford University Press, 1925); Michael Bliss, *William Osler: A Life in Medicine* (New York: Oxford University Press, 1999). For contemporary knowledge on the epidemiology and pathophysiology of syphilis, see G. P. Garnett et al., "The Natural History of Syphilis: Implications for the Transmission Dynamics and Control of Infection," *Sexually Transmitted Diseases* 24 (1997): 185–200; Institute of Medicine, *The Hidden Epidemic: Confronting Sexually Transmitted Diseases*, ed. T. R. Eng and W. T. Butler (Washington, D.C.: National Academy Press, 1997). For historical background, see Quétel, *History of Syphilis;* Ludwig Fleck, *Genesis and Development of a Scientific Fact* (Chicago: University of Chicago Press, 1979); Allan Brandt, *No Magic Bullet: A Social History of Venereal Disease in the United States Since 1880* (New York: Oxford University Press, 1987).

23. "Pneumocystis Pneumonia, Los Angeles," *Morbidity and Mortality Weekly Report* (MMWR), June 5, 1981, pp. 250–52; "Kaposi's Sarcoma and *Pneumocystis pneumonia* Among Homosexual Men—New York and California," *MMWR*, July 3, 1981, pp. 305–8; "Opportunistic Infections and Kaposi's Sarcoma Among Haitians in the United States," *MMWR*, July 9, 1982, pp. 353–54, 360–61; *"Pneumocystis carinii* Pneumonia Among Persons with Hemophilia A," *MMWR*, July 16, 1982, pp. 365–67; "Possible Transfusion Acquired Immune Deficiency Syndrome (AIDS)—California," *MMWR*, Dec. 10, 1982, pp. 652–54; Kent Sepkowitz, "AIDS: The First Twenty Years," *New England Journal of Medicine* 344 (2001): 1764–72; For a summary of the media coverage of the early years of the AIDS epidemic, see James Kinsella, *Covering the Plague: AIDS and the American Media* (New Brunswick, N.J.: Rutgers University Press, 1989), pp. 9–10.

24. Ronald Bayer and Gerald Oppenheimer, *AIDS Doctors: Voices from the Epidemic: An Oral History* (New York: Oxford University Press, 2000), pp. 33–34.

25. Hughes Evans, "The Discovery of Child Sexual Abuse in America," in *Formative Years: Children's Health in America, 1880–2000*, ed. Alexandra Stern and Howard Markel (Ann Arbor: University of Michigan Press, 2002), pp. 243–44.

26. Susan Little et al., "Antiretroviral-Drug Resistance Among Patients Recently Infected with HIV," *New England Journal of Medicine* 347 (2002): 385–94; Martin Hirsch, "HIV Drug Resistance—A Chink in the Armor," *New England Journal of Medicine* 347 (2002): 438–39; Anthony Fauci, "Multifactorial Nature of Human Immunodeficiency Virus Disease: Implications for Therapy," *Science* 262 (1993): 1011–18; Fauci et al., "Immunopathogenic Mechanisms of HIV Infection," *Annals of Internal Medicine* 124 (1996): 654–63; P. T. Cohen, "Understanding HIV Disease: Hallmarks, Clinical Spectrum, and What We Need to Know," in *The AIDS Knowledge Base*, 3rd ed., ed. P. T. Cohen et al. (Philadelphia: Lippincott, Williams and Wilkins, 1999), pp. 175–94; J. M. Kilby and M. S. Saag, "Natural History of HIV-1 Disease," in *Textbook of AIDS Medicine*, 2nd ed., ed. T. C. Merigan, J. G. Bartlett, and D. Bolognesi (Baltimore: Williams and Wilkins, 1999),

pp. 49–58; Montagnier, *Virus;* Linqi Zhang et al., "Contribution of Human Alpha-Defensin-1, -2, -3 to the Anti-HIV-I Activity of CD8 Antiviral Factor," *Science* 298 (2002): 995–1000.

27. John Crewdson, *Science Fictions: A Scientific Mystery, A Massive Cover-Up, and the Dark Legacy of Robert Gallo* (Boston: Little, Brown, 2002); Montagnier, *Virus;* Robert Gallo, *Virus Hunting: AIDS, Cancer, and the Human Retrovirus: A Story of Scientific Discovery* (New York: Basic Books, 1991).

28. Shilts, *And the Band Played On,* pp. 71, 78, 86–87; Grmek, *History of AIDS,* pp. 15–16; James Goedert et al., "Amyl Nitrate May Alter T Lymphocytes in Homosexual Men," *Lancet* 1 (1982): 412–16. Despite an enormous amount of investigative work, no significant correlation between the use (or abuse) of amyl (or butyl) nitrate and AIDS has been demonstrated. See, for example, M. Marmor et al., "Kaposi's Sarcoma in Homosexual Men," *Annals of Internal Medicine* 100 (1984): 809–15; Harold Jaffe et al., "National Case-Control Study of Kaposi's Sarcoma and *Pneumocystis Carinii* Pneumonia in Homosexual Men: Part 1: Epidemiologic Results," *Annals of Internal Medicine* 99 (1983): 145–51; James Goedert et al., "Effect of T4 Count and Co-factors on the Incidence of AIDS in Homosexual Men," *Journal of the American Medical Association* 257 (1987): 331–34; B. F. Polk et al., "Predictors of the Acquired Immunodeficiency Syndrome Developing in a Cohort of Seropositive Homosexual Men," *New England Journal of Medicine* 316 (1987): 61–66.

29. Heinl and Heinl, *Written in Blood,* pp. 685–87; L. B. Moskowitz et al., "Unusual Causes of Death in Haitians Residing in Miami: High Prevalence of Opportunistic Infections," *Journal of the American Medical Association* 250 (1983): 1187–91; A. E. Pitchenik et al., "Tuberculosis, Atypical Mycobacteriosis, and the Acquired Immunodeficiency Syndrome Among Haitian and Non-Haitian Patients in South Florida," *Annals of Internal Medicine* 101 (1984): 641–45; Farmer, *AIDS and Accusation,* pp. 121–33.

30. Jean Pape et al., "Characteristics of the Acquired Immunodeficiency Syndrome (AIDS) in Haiti," *New England Journal of Medicine* 309 (1983): 945–50; Pape et al., "Acquired Immunodeficiency Syndrome in Haiti," *Clinical Research* 32, no. 2 (1984): 379; Pape et al., "The Acquired Immunodeficiency Syndrome in Haiti," *Annals of Internal Medicine* 103 (1985): 674–78; Pape et al., "Risk Factors Associated with AIDS in Haiti," *American Journal of Medical Science* 291, no. 1 (1986): 4–7.

31. Farmer, *AIDS and Accusation,* pp. 196–201, 220–26, 237–38.

32. "AIDS Update," *MMWR,* June 24, 1983, pp. 309–11. See also "Opportunistic Infections and Kaposi's Sarcoma Among Haitians in the United States," *MMWR,* July 9, 1982, pp. 353–61.

33. H. M. Smith, "AIDS: The Haitian Connection," *MD* 27, no. 12 (1983): 46–52; *Washington Post,* Aug. 2, 1983, p. A1; R. Sabatier, *Blaming Others: Prejudice, Race and Worldwide AIDS* (Washington, D.C.: Panos Institute, 1988), p. 45.

34. Gerald M. Oppenheimer, "In the Eye of the Storm: The Epidemiological Construction of AIDS," in *AIDS: The Burdens of History,* ed. Elizabeth Fee and Daniel M. Fox (Berkeley: University of California Press, 1988), pp. 267–300.

35. Steven Nachman and G. Dreyfuss, "Haitians and AIDS in South Florida," *Medical Anthropology Quarterly* 17, no. 2 (1986): 32–33.

36. Sabatier, *Blaming Others,* pp. 46–47; Shilts, *And the Band Played On,* p. 322; Farmer, *AIDS and Accusation,* pp. 213–20.

37. *Miami Herald,* Aug. 20, 1983, p. B1. See also *Miami News,* May 30, 1983, p. A5.

38. Smith, "AIDS: The Haitian Connection," p. 46.

39. *Boston Globe,* May 11, 1990, p. 25.

40. Barbara Sanon, "4.20.90: Proud of Our Blood," *Poz Magazine,* April 2000, p. 72.

41. *New York Times,* Mar. 14, 1990, p. A20.

42. *Haiti-Progrès,* April 25–May 1, 1990, p. 13. See also *New York Times,* Apr. 21, 1990, p. A10.

43. *New York Daily News,* Apr. 25, 1990, p. 23. See also *Haiti-Progrès,* May 24–30, 1995, p. 1.

44. *New York Times,* Apr. 29, 1990, sec. 4, p. 20.

45. Sanon, "4.20.90," p. 72.

46. Catanese, *Haitians,* pp. 1–5; Laguerre, *American Odyssey,* pp. 21–32; J. Dreyfuss, "The Invisible Immigrants," *New York Times Magazine,* May 23, 1993, pp. 20–21, 80–82.

47. Jean-Bertrand Aristide, *In the Parish of the Poor: Writings from Haiti* (New York: Orbis, 1990), p. 67. In 1994 Aristide was briefly returned to power by the U.S. military occupation in Haiti. He again became president in late 2000.

48. George H. W. Bush, President, "Interdiction of Illegal Aliens, Executive Order #12,807," *Federal Register* 57, no. 105 (May 24, 1992): 23133–34. During this period a far more infamous quarantine against AIDS was enacted in Cuba proper. See, for example, Nancy Scheper-Hughes, "AIDS, Public Health and Human Rights in Cuba," *Lancet* 342 (1993): 966; Tim Golden, "Patients Pay a High Price in Cuba's War on AIDS," *New York Times,* Oct. 16, 1995, p. A1.

49. *Chicago Tribune,* June 22, 1993, sec. 1, p. 4; *Los Angeles Times,* June 22, 1993, p. A1; *Washington Post,* June 22, 1993, p. A1; *Washington Times,* June 22, 1993, p. A1; *New York Newsday,* June 22, 1993, p. 7.

50. "God and Country Presents GTMO's Haitian Invasion: The Day We Bit Off a Little More Than We Could Chew," http://www.angelfire.com/va/godandcountry/haitian.html. Accessed Sept. 10, 2003.

51. Ibid.

52. Ibid.

53. See, for example, *New York Times,* June 9, 1993, p. B9.

54. Paul Farmer, *The Uses of Haiti* (Monroe, Maine: Common Courage Press, 1994), p. 264; see also Farmer, *Pathologies of Power: Health, Human Rights, and the New War on the Poor* (Berkeley: University of California Press, 2003), pp. 51–90.

55. *New York Times,* Dec. 10, 1992, p. A13; *Washington Post,* Dec. 11, 1992, p. A1.

56. Farmer, *Uses of Haiti,* pp. 277–85.

57. *San Francisco Chronicle,* Aug. 31, 1992, p. 1; Farmer, *Uses of Haiti,* pp. 279–80.

58. *The Nation,* Jan. 4–11, 1993, p. 5.

59. Christine Gorman, "Opening the Borders to AIDS," *Time,* Feb. 22, 1993, p. 45.

60. *New York Times,* Dec. 10, 1992, p. A13.

61. Gorman, "Opening the Borders to AIDS," p. 45.

62. *Congressional Record,* 103rd Congr., 1st sess., U.S. Senate, Feb. 17, 1993, p. 2865.

63. J. Price, "Dropping AIDS Ban Irks Doctors," *Washington Times,* Feb. 10, 1993, p. A1.

64. House of Representatives, *Congressional Record,* 103rd Congr., 1st sess., Mar. 11, 1993, p. 4764.

65. National Institutes of Health Revitalization Act of 1993, pub. 1, no. 103–143, sec. 2007, 107 stat. 210, codified as amended at U.S.C., sec. 1182, (a) (1) (A) (I), supplement 1993; G. J. Annas, "Detention of HIV-Positive Haitians at Guantánamo," *New England Journal of Medicine* 329 (1993): 589–92; K. A. Krzynowek, "*Haitian Centers Council, Inc.* v. *Sale:* Rejecting the Indefinite Detention of HIV-Infected Aliens," *Journal of Contemporary Health Law and Policy* 11 (1995): 541–62; A. L. Fairchild and E. A. Tynan, "Policies of Containment: Immigration in the Era of AIDS," *American Journal of Public Health* 84 (1994): 2011–22. For a summary of contemporary quarantine and immigrant medical inspection regulations of the USPHS, see U.S. Department of Health and Human Services, *Public Health Screening at U.S. Ports of Entry: A Guide for Federal Inspectors,* rev. ed. (Washington, D.C.: U.S. Government Printing Office, 1996). For HIV incidence data during this period, see J. M. Karon et al., "Prevalence of HIV Infection in the United States, 1984 to 1992," *Journal of the American Medical Association* 276 (1996): 126–31.

66. *New York Times,* Mar. 27, 1993, p. A9.

67. *New York Times,* June 9, 1993, p. B4; *Haitian Centers Council* v. *Sale,* 823 F. Suppl. 1028 (E.D.N.Y. 1993).

68. *New York Times,* June 10, 1993, p. A12.

69. *New York Times,* June 13, 1993, p. A24.

70. *New York Times,* June 15, 1993, p. A20.

71. *New York Times,* May 25, 1998, p. A1.

72. UNAIDS/World Health Organization, *AIDS Epidemic Update,* December 2003 (Geneva: Joint United Nations Programme on HIV/AIDS, 2003); Robert Steinbrook, "Beyond Barcelona: The Global Response to HIV," *New England Journal of Medicine* 347 (2002): 553–54; Fitzhugh Mullan, "Purple Is the Color of the Future," *Health Affairs* 21 (2002): 215–20.

73. Lawrence Altman, "AIDS in Five Nations Called Security Threat," *New York Times,* Oct. 1, 2002, p. A10; Geoff Dyer, "CIA Warns of New Frontiers in AIDS Epidemic," *Financial Times,* Oct. 4, 2002, p. 10.

CHAPTER SIX • SOUNDING THE CHOLERA ALARM IN DETROIT

1. Olivier Zunz, *The Changing Face of Inequality: Urbanization, Industrial Development and Immigrants in Detroit, 1880–1920* (Chicago: University of Chicago Press, 1982); Thomas Sugrue, *The Origins of the Urban Crisis: Race and Inequality in Postwar Detroit* (Princeton: Princeton University Press, 1996); Ze'ev Chafets, *Devil's Night and Other True Tales of Detroit* (New York: Random House, 1990).

2. Detroit was a well-known station along the actual Underground Railroad that transported fugitive slaves in the decades before the Civil War. Called the "Midnight" station, it was the last point before Canada, and between 1831 and 1865 more than 40,000 slaves proceeded along this path. See Henrietta Buckmaster, *Let My People Go: The Story of the Underground Railroad and the Growth of the Abolition Movement* (Boston: Beacon, 1941); Levi Coffin, *Reminiscences of Levi Coffin, the Reputed President of the Underground Railroad* (New York: Arno, 1968).

3. See, for example, Nancy Foner, *From Ellis Island to JFK: New York's Two Great Waves of Immigration* (New Haven: Yale University Press, 2000).

4. Lillian Wald, *The House on Henry Street* (New York: Holt, 1915), and *Windows on Henry Street* (Boston: Little, Brown, 1934).

5. Jane Addams, *Twenty Years at Hull-House, with Autobiographical Notes* (New York: Macmillan, 1910), and *The Second Twenty Years at Hull-House, September 1909–September 1929* (New York: Macmillan, 1930); Mary Kingsbury Simkhovitch, *Neighborhood: My Story of Greenwich House* (New York: Norton, 1938).

6. Brian Leigh Dunnigan, *Frontier Metropolis: Picturing Early Detroit, 1701–1838* (Detroit: Wayne State University Press, 2001).

7. Arthur Woodford, *This Is Detroit, 1701–2001* (Detroit: Wayne State University Press, 2001).

8. The other founders were a Protestant minister named John Monteith and a prominent lawyer and judge named Augustus Woodward. Howard Peckham, *The Making of the University of Michigan, 1817–1992* (Ann Arbor: Bentley Historical Library/University of Michigan, 1994).

9. Leslie Teutler, "Gabriel Richard," *American National Biography,* vol. 18 (New York: Oxford University Press, 1999), pp. 433–34; Charles Rosenberg, *The Cholera Years: The United States in 1832, 1849, and 1866* (Chicago: University of Chicago Press, 1987).

10. Owsei Temkin, "An Historical Analysis of the Concept of Infection," in his *The Double Face of Janus and Other Essays in the History of Medicine* (Baltimore: Johns Hopkins University Press, 1977). See also Nancy Tomes, *The Gospel of Germs: Men, Women and the Microbe in American Life* (Cambridge: Harvard University Press, 1998); Charles E. A. Winslow, *The Conquest of Epidemic Disease: A Chapter in the History of Ideas* (New York: Hafner, 1967).

11. See, for example, Victor Safford, *Immigration Problems: Personal Experiences of an Official* (New York: Dodd, Mead, 1925); "Report on the Sweating System," U.S. House of Representatives, Feb. 13, 1892, *Congressional Record,* pp. H181–H200. See also Daniel Bender, "Inspecting Workers: Medical Examination, Labor Organizing, and the Evidence of Sexual Difference," *Radical History Review* 80 (2001): 51–75, and "A Hero . . . for the Weak: Work, Consumption, and the Enfeebled Jewish Worker, 1881–1924," *International Labor and Working-Class History* 56 (1999): 1–22.

12. "Instructing Foreign Parents and Children," *School Health News: Published Monthly for the Information of School Teachers by the Bureau of Public Health Education, New York City Department of Health,* January 1921, p. 5.

13. All of the subsequent quotes attributed to immigrants at Freedom House in this chapter were transcribed by the author and logged in a journal entitled "Freedom House Diaries."

14. Philip Gourevitch, *We wish to inform you that tomorrow we will be killed with our families: Stories from Rwanda* (New York: Picador USA/Farrar, Straus and Giroux, 1998), pp. 47–48.

15. Fergal Keane, *Season of Blood: A Rwandan Journey* (London: Penguin USA, 1997).

16. Gerard Prunier, *The Rwanda Crisis: History of a Genocide* (New York: Columbia University Press, 1997).

17. African Rights Organization, *Rwanda: Death, Despair and Defiance* (London: African Rights Organization, 1994).

18. For general accounts of this practice, see Sylvester Monroe, "Hot Ticket: First-Class Problem," *Time*, Mar. 15, 1999, p. 71; Jeff Goodell, "How to Fake a Passport," *New York Times Magazine*, Feb. 10, 2002, pp. 44–49.

19. See, for example, *New York Times*, July 21, 1994, pp. A1, A8; July 22, 1994, pp. A1, A11; July 24, 1994, p. A1; July 25, 1994, p. A7; July 26, 1994, p. A6; July 27, 1994, p. A11; July 28, 1994, p. A1; Aug. 1, 1994, p. A3; Aug. 2, 1994, p. A20; Aug. 5, 1994, p. A6; Nov. 7, 1996, p. A12; Apr. 5, 1997, p. A1; Apr. 13, 1997, p. A1; Apr. 25, 1997, p. A6; Goma Epidemiology Group, "Public Health Impact of Rwandan Refugee Crisis: What Happened in Goma, Zaire, in July, 1994?" *Lancet* 345 (1995): 339–44; D. L. Swerdlow and O. Levine, "Cholera Control Among Rwandan Refugees in Zaire," *Lancet* 344 (1994): 1302–3. Zaire was the former name of the Democratic Republic of the Congo.

20. Paul Farmer, *Infections and Inequalities: The Modern Plagues* (Berkeley: University of California Press, 2001); David Satcher, "Emerging Infections: Getting Ahead of the Curve," *Emerging Infectious Diseases* 1, no. 1 (1995): 1–6.

21. There are a great many studies on the history of cholera, including Rosenberg, *The Cholera Years;* Howard Markel, *Quarantine!: East European Jewish Immigrants and the New York City Epidemics of 1892* (Baltimore: Johns Hopkins University Press, 1997); Richard Evans, *Death in Hamburg: Society and Politics in the Cholera Years, 1830–1910* (New York: Oxford University Press, 1987); R. J. Morris, *Cholera, 1832: The Social Response to an Epidemic* (New York: Holmes and Meier, 1976); M. Durey, *The Return of the Plague: British Society and the Cholera, 1831–1832* (Dublin: Gill and Macmillan, 1979); François Delaporte, *Disease and Civilization: The Cholera in Paris, 1832,* trans. Arthur Goldhammer (Cambridge: MIT Press, 1986); C. J. Kudlick, *Cholera in Post-Revolutionary Paris: A Cultural History* (Berkeley: University of California Press, 1996); M. Pelling, *Cholera, Fever, and English Medicine, 1825–1865* (Oxford, Eng.: Oxford University Press, 1978); R. E. McGrew, *Russia and the Cholera, 1823–1832* (Madison: University of Wisconsin Press, 1965); N. Longmate, *King Cholera: The Biography of a Disease* (London: Hamish Hamilton, 1966); F. Snowden, *Naples in the Time of Cholera, 1884–1911* (New York: Cambridge University Press, 1995); J. S. Chambers, *The Conquest of Cholera: America's Greatest Scourge* (New York: Macmillan, 1938); Christopher Meehan and Howard Markel, "Cholera, Historical," in *Encyclopedia of Microbiology,* ed. Joshua Lederberg, vol. 1 (San Diego: Academic Press, 2000), pp. 155–61.

22. "The Kind of 'Assisted Emigrant' We Can Not Afford to Admit," *Puck Magazine*, July 18, 1883, p. 324.

23. John Snow, *Snow on Cholera, Being a Reprint of Two Papers* (New York: Hafner, 1965).

24. K. Bryn Thomas, "John Snow," *Dictionary of Scientific Biography*, vol. 12 (New York: Scribner's, 1973), pp. 502–3.

25. Edward O. Shakespeare, *Report on Cholera in Europe and India* (Washington, D.C.: U.S. Government Printing Office, 1890), pp. 21–43. See Edmund Wendt, ed., *A Treatise on Asiatic Cholera* (New York: William C. Wood, 1885), pp. 61–68; Robert Koch, "An Address on Cholera and Its Bacillus Read Before the Imperial German Board of Health at Berlin," *British Medical Journal* 2 (1884): 403–7; Claude E. Dolman, "Robert Koch," in *Dictionary of Scientific Biography*, vol. 7 (New York: Scribner's, 1973), pp. 420–33; Lester King, "Dr. Koch's Postulates," *Journal of the History of Medicine and Allied Sciences* 7 (1952): 350–61; Robert Koch, *Essays of Robert Koch*, trans. K. C. Carter (New York: Greenwood, 1987).

26. Sherwin Nuland, "Hate in the Time of Cholera," *The New Republic*, May 26, 1997, pp. 32–37; Nuland, *Lost in America: A Journey with My Father* (New York: Knopf, 2003), p. 56.

27. Joseph Stein, Jerry Bock, and Sheldon Harnick, *Fiddler on the Roof* (New York: Crown, 1964).

28. Eugene F. Gangarosa et al., "The Nature of the Gastrointestinal Lesion in Asiatic Cholera and Its Relation to Pathogenesis: A Biopsy Study," *American Journal of Tropical Medicine and Hygiene* 9 (1960): 125–35.

29. Dhiman Barua and William B. Greenough, eds., *Cholera* (New York: Plenum, 1992); C. C. J. Carpenter et al., "Clinical Studies in Asiatic Cholera," *Bulletin of the Johns Hopkins Hospital* 118 (1966): 165–245. Cholera's genomic sequence has recently been mapped out, enabling scientists to better understand both its history and the ways and means to prevent another outbreak. See J. F. Heidelberg et al., "DNA Sequence of Both Chromosomes of the Cholera Pathogen, *Vibrio cholerae*," *Nature* 406 (2000): 477–83; Matthew Waldor and Debabrata Raychaudhuri, "Bacterial Genomics: Treasure Trove for Cholera Research," *Nature* 406 (2000): 469–70; Barry Bloom, "On the Particularity of Pathogens," *Nature* 406 (2000): 760–61.

30. Evans, *Death in Hamburg*, p. 230.

31. "Cholera," *World Health Organization Report on Global Surveillance of Epidemic-Prone Infectious Diseases*, 2001, http://www.who.int/csr/resources/publications/surveillance/en/cholera.pdf. Accessed Nov. 13, 2003.

32. Jamie Pittock, "More Pipes Won't Solve the World's Water Crisis: The Johannesburg Summit," *International Herald Tribune*, Aug. 13, 2002, p. 4.

33. William Welch, "Asiatic Cholera in Its Relations to Sanitary Reforms," in *Papers and Addresses by William Henry Welch*, vol. 1 (Baltimore: Johns Hopkins University Press, 1920), pp. 599–606. Quote is from p. 605.

34. "Laboratory-Based Surveillance for Rotavirus in the United States, July 1996 to June 1997," *Mortality and Morbidity Weekly Report* 46 (1997) 1092–94; R. I. Glass et al., "The Epidemiology of Rotavirus Diarrhea in the United States: Surveillance and Estimates of Disease Burden," *Journal of Infectious Disease* 174, supplement 1

(1996): S5–S11; I. De Zoysa and F. G. Feachem, "Interventions for the Control of Diarrhoeal Diseases Among Young Children: Rotavirus and Cholera Immunization," *Bulletin of the World Health Organization* 63 (1985): 569–83.

EPILOGUE • "PUBLIC HEALTH IS PURCHASABLE"

1. Hermann Biggs, "Public Health Is Purchasable," *Monthly Bulletin of the Department of Health of the City of New York,* Oct. 11, 1911, pp. 225–26. Quote is from p. 226.

2. Simon Flexner and James Thomas Flexner, *William Henry Welch and the Heroic Age of American Medicine* (New York: Viking, 1941), p. 119. Biggs recalled Welch's lecture and demonstration as "my first inspiration."

3. William Welch, foreword to Charles E. A. Winslow, *The Life of Hermann M. Biggs, M.D., D.Sc., LL.D.: Physician and Statesman of the Public Health* (Philadelphia: Lea and Febiger, 1929), p. xii. In addition to this fine biography of Biggs and his contributions to American public health, see Howard Markel, "Hermann Michael Biggs," in *American National Biography,* ed. John A. Garraty and Mark C. Carnes, vol. 2 (New York: Oxford University Press, 1999), pp. 759–60; Markel, *Quarantine!: East European Jewish Immigrants and the New York City Epidemics of 1892* (Baltimore: Johns Hopkins University Press, 1997), pp. 105–7, 125–29, 158–61.

4. Abraham Cahan. "Bourgeoisie and the Cholera" (editorial), *New York Arbeiter Zeitung,* Sept. 26, 1892, pp. 2, 1.

5. Prabhat Jha et al., "Improving the Health of the Global Poor," *Science* 295 (2002): 2036–39; Caroline Ash and Barbara Jasny, "Unmet Needs in Public Health," *Science* 295 (2002): 2035; David Bloom and David Canning, "The Health and Wealth of Nations," *Science* 287 (2000): 1207–9; Paul Farmer, *Infections and Inequalities: The Modern Plagues* (Berkeley: University of California Press, 2001); Howard Markel and Stephen Doyle, "The Epidemic Scorecard," *New York Times,* Apr. 30, 2003, p. A31.

6. Paul Ewald, *Evolution of Infectious Disease* (New York: Oxford University Press, 1994), and *Plague Time: The New Germ Theory of Disease* (New York: Anchor Books/Random House, 2002); Joshua Lederberg, Robert Shope, and Stanley Oakes, *Emerging Infections: Microbial Threats to Health in the United States* (Washington, D.C.: National Academy Press, 1992); U.S. National Intelligence Council, *The Global Infectious Disease Threat and Its Implications for the United States,* NIE 99-17D, January 2000, http://www.cia.gov/cia/reports/nie/report/nie99-17d.html. Accessed Nov. 15, 2003.

7. See, for example, Albert Camus, *The Plague* (New York: Vintage, 1991); Charles Rosenberg, "What Is an Epidemic?: AIDS in Historical Perspective," in *Explaining Epidemics and Other Studies in the History of Medicine,* ed. Rosenberg (New York: Cambridge University Press, 1992), pp. 278–92.

8. Laurie Garrett, *Betrayal of Trust: The Collapse of Global Public Health* (New York: Hyperion, 2000), p. 557, and *The Coming Plague: Newly Emerging Diseases in a World Out of Balance* (New York: Farrar, Straus and Giroux, 1994).

9. Garrett, *Betrayal of Trust,* pp. 545–85; Jordan Kassalow, *Why Health Is Important to U.S. Foreign Policy* (New York: Council on Foreign Relations/Milbank Memorial Fund, 2001); Denise Grady, "Bioterror Agents Join List of 'Emerging' Ills," *New York Times,* Apr. 2, 2002, p. D1.

10. United Nations Development Programme, Millennium Development Goals, http://www.undp.org/mdg/. Accessed Nov. 6, 2003.

11. At present, the World Bank defines high-income countries as those where the annual per capita income is more than $9,266. In low-income countries, the annual per capita income is $755 or less. See Jeffrey Sachs, "Investing in Health for Economic Development," *Project Syndicate,* January 2002, http://www.project-syndicate.org. Accessed Nov. 6, 2003.

12. Sachs, "Investing in Health"; Sachs, "Helping the World's Poorest," *The Economist* 352 (Aug. 20, 1999): 17–20; Barry Bloom et al., "Investing in the World Health Organization," *Science* 284 (1999): 911; Sachs, A. D. Mellinger, and J. L. Gallup, "The Geography of Poverty and Wealth," *Scientific American* 284, no. 3 (2001): 70–75; Andrew Price-Smith, *The Health of Nations: Infectious Disease, Environmental Change, and Their Effects on National Security and Development* (Cambridge: MIT Press, 2002). For data on low-, middle-, and high-income nations in the world today, see http://www.worldbank.org/data/databytopic/databytopic.html. Accessed Nov. 13, 2003.

13. Ash and Jasny, "Unmet Needs in Public Health," p. 2035; Jha et al., "Improving the Health of the Global Poor," pp. 2036–39; Bloom and Canning, "Health and Wealth of Nations," pp. 1207–9; J. L. Gallup and J. D. Sachs, "The Economic Burden of Malaria," *American Journal of Tropical Medicine and Hygiene* 64, 1–2 suppl. (2001): 85–96.

INDEX

THE HOT ZONE
*A Terrifying True Story*
by Richard Preston

*The Hot Zone* tells the dramatic true story of when a highly infectious, deadly virus from central Africa suddenly appeared in the suburbs of Washington, D.C. In a few days 90 percent of its victims were dead. A secret military SWAT team of soldiers and scientists was mobilized to stop the outbreak of this exotic "hot" virus.

Science/0-385-49522-6

A FIELD GUIDE TO GERMS
by Wayne Biddle

In *A Field Guide to Germs*, Wayne Biddle brings readers face-to-face with one hundred of the best-known pathogens that live in and around us. From cholera to chlamydia, TB to HIV, rabies to Congo-Crimean encephalitis, anthrax to Zika fever, and back to good old rhinitis (the common cold), this book is both a reference and a fascinating look at the astonishing impact of microorganisms on history.

Science/1-4000-3051-X

PLAGUE TIME
*The New Germ Theory of Disease*
by Paul W. Ewald

In this eye-opening exploration, Ewald argues against convention that germs appear to be at the root of heart disease, Alzheimer's, and other chronic diseases, these often-ignored agents cause long-term infections, and new evolutionary theories can both reveal how germs function and offer opportunities for controlling modern plagues.

Health/Medicine/0-385-72184-6

BIOGRAPHY OF A GERM
by Arno Karlen

*Borrelia burgdorferi* is the germ that causes Lyme disease. Exploring its evolution, its daily existence, and its journey from ticks to mice to deer to humans, Karlen lucidly examines the life and world of this recently prominent germ. He also describes how it attacks the human body, and how by changing the environment, people are now much more likely to come into contact with it.

Science/Biology/0-385-72066-1

### HOW WE DIE
*Reflections on Life's Final Chapter*
by Sherwin B. Nuland

In this National Book award–winning book, the distinguished surgeon Sherwin B. Nuland describes the mechanisms of cancer, heart attack, stroke, AIDS, and Alzheimer's disease with clinical exactness and poetic elegance—with the sensitivity of a man recalling his own intimate losses. Even as Nuland dispels the myth of the dignified death (and decries the technical hubris of modern medicine), he succeeds in restoring death to its ancient place in human existence.

Medicine/0-679-74244-1

### VIRUS HUNTER
*Thirty Years of Battling Hot Viruses Around the World*
by C. J. Peters and Mark Olshaker

Dr. C. J. Peters has been on the front lines of our biological battle against "hot" viruses around the world for three decades. He has learned countless lessons about out interspecies turf wars with infectious agents. Because of new, emerging viruses, and the return of old, "vanquished" ones for which vaccines do not exist, there remains a very real danger of a new epidemic that could, without proper surveillance and early intervention, spread worldwide virtually overnight.

Autobiography/Science/0-385-48558-1

### WHY WE GET SICK
*The New Science of Darwinian Medicine*
by Randolph M. Nesse and George C. Williams

The next time you get sick, consider this before you pick up the aspirin: your body may be doing exactly what it's supposed to. In this groundbreaking book, two pioneers of the emerging science of Darwinian medicine argue that illness as well as factors that predispose us toward it are subject to the same laws of natural selection that otherwise make our bodies such miracles of design.

Science/Medicine/0-679-74674-9

VINTAGE AND ANCHOR BOOKS
Available from your local bookstore, or call toll-free to order:
1-800-793-2665 (credit cards only).